T0261558

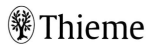

Direct Diagnosis in Radiology

Musculoskeletal Imaging

Maximilian Reiser, MD, Dr hc
Professor of Radiology
Head of Department of Clinical Radiology
University of Munich-Grosshadern Campus
Munich, Germany

Andrea Baur-Melnyk, MD
Section Chief
Associate Professor of Radiology
Department of Clinical Radiology
University of Munich-Grosshadern Campus
Munich, Germany

Christian Glaser, MD
Supervising Physician and Section Chief MRI
Consultant MSK Imaging
Department of Clinical Radiology
University of Munich-Grosshadern Campus
Munich, Germany

355 Illustrations

Thieme
Stuttgart · New York

Library of Congress Cataloging-in-Publication Data

Reiser, Maximilian.
    [Bewegungsapparat. English]
    Musculoskeletal imaging / Maximilian Reiser, Andrea Baur-Melnyk, Christian Glaser ; [translator, Stephanie Kramer].
        p. ; cm. – (Direct diagnosis in radiology)
    Includes bibliographical references.
    ISBN 978-3-13-145161-3 (TPS, rest of world : alk. paper) – ISBN 978-1-60406-085-0 (TPN, the Americas : alk. paper) 1. Musculoskeletal system–Imaging–Handbooks, manuals, etc. 2. Musculoskeletal system–Diseases–Diagnosis–Handbooks, manuals, etc. I. Baur-Melnyk, Andrea. II. Glaser, Christian. III. Title. IV. Series.
    [DNLM: 1. Musculoskeletal Diseases–diagnosis–Handbooks. 2. Musculoskeletal ystem–radiography–Handbooks.
    3. Diagnosis, Differential–Handbooks.
    4. Diagnostic Imaging–Handbooks.
    WE 39 R375b 2007a]
        RC925.7.R4513 2008
        616.7'07572–dc22   2007045999

This book is an authorized and revised translation of the German edition published and copyrighted 2007 by Georg Thieme Verlag, Stuttgart, Germany. Title of the German edition: Pareto-Reihe Radiologie: Bewegungsapparat.

Translator: Stephanie Kramer, BA, Dipl Trans, IoL, Berlin, Germany

Illustrator: Markus Voll, Munich, Germany

© 2008 Georg Thieme Verlag KG
Rüdigerstraße 14, 70469 Stuttgart, Germany
http://www.thieme.de
Thieme New York, 333 Seventh Avenue,
New York, NY 10001, USA
http://www.thieme.com

Cover design: Thieme Publishing Group
Typesetting by Ziegler + Müller, Kirchentellinsfurt, Germany
Printed by APPL aprinta Druck, Wemding, Germany

ISBN 978-3-13-145161-3
                    1 2 3 4 5 6

Important note: Medicine is an ever-changing science undergoing continual development. Research and clinical experience are continually expanding our knowledge, in particular our knowledge of proper treatment and drug therapy. Insofar as this book mentions any dosage or application, readers may rest assured that the authors, editors, and publishers have made every effort to ensure that such references are in accordance with **the state of knowledge at the time of production of the book.**

Nevertheless, this does not involve, imply, or express any guarantee or responsibility on the part of the publishers in respect to any dosage instructions and forms of applications stated in the book. **Every user is requested to examine carefully** the manufacturers' leaflets accompanying each drug and to check, if necessary in consultation with a physician or specialist, whether the dosage schedules mentioned therein or the contraindications stated by the manufacturers differ from the statements made in the present book. Such examination is particularly important with drugs that are either rarely used or have been newly released on the market. Every dosage schedule or every form of application used is entirely at the user's own risk and responsibility. The authors and publishers request every user to report to the publishers any discrepancies or inaccuracies noticed. If errors in this work are found after publication, errata will be posted at www.thieme.com on the product description page.

Special thanks go to Maria Triantafyllou and Julia Dinges,
who assisted in preparing the manuscript.
For valuable insights into the clinical aspects of the pathologies
presented in this work, we would like to thank Christof Birkenmaier, MD,
and Stefan Piltz, MD, Associate Professor of Radiology.

Contents

ACJ	acromioclavicular joint	**MFH**	malignant fibrous histiocytoma
ACR	American College of Radiology	**MIP**	maximum intensity projection
ACT	autologous chondrocyte transplantation	**MRI**	magnetic resonance imaging
ALPSA	anterior labroligamentous periosteal sleeve avulsion	**MSCT**	multislice CT
AOT	autologous osteochondral transplantation	**MTP**	metatarsophalangeal (joint)
AP	anteroposterior	**NOF**	nonossifying fibroma
AP	alkaline phosphatase	**NSAID**	nonsteroidal anti-inflammatory drug
ARCO	Association Research Circulation Osseous	**OATS**	osteochondral allograft transport system
T	thoracic vertebra	**OTA**	Orthopaedic Trauma Association
CISS	constructive interference in steady state	**PA**	posteroanterior
CRMO	chronic recurrent multifocal osteomyelitis	**PBNS**	pigmented villonodular synovitis
CRP	C-reactive protein	**PET**	positron emission tomography
CRPS	complex regional pain syndrome	**PIP**	proximal interphalangeal (joint)
DIP	distal interphalangeal (joint)	**POEMS**	polyneuropathy, organomegaly, endocrinopathy, M-protein band skin
DISH	diffuse idiopathic skeletal hyperostosis	**PTH**	parathormone
DTPA	diethylenetriaminepenta-acetic acid	**QCT**	quantitative CT
DXA	dual-energy X-ray absorptiometry	**SE**	spin echo
		SI	sacroiliac
ESR	erythrocyte sedimentation rate	**SLAP**	superior labrum anterior to posterior (lesion)
GE	gradient echo	**TNF**	tumor necrosis factor
GLAD	glenolabral articular disruption	**STIR**	short tau inversion recovery
HLA	human leukocyte antigen	**TSE**	turbo spin echo
HU	Hounsfield unit	**UVA**	ultraviolet A
IPJ	interphalangeal (joint)	**WE**	water excitation
MCP	metacarpophalangeal (joint)	**WHO**	World Health Organization
MEN	multiple endocrine neoplasia		

Definition
....

▶ **Epidemiology**
Exact incidence unknown since lesions often asymptomatic (especially medullary osteomas) ● In an estimated 10% of all patients osteomas are found incidentally in the pelvis, vertebral bodies, proximal femur (intertrochanteric location/femoral neck), or ribs; in 1% in the paranasal sinuses ● Parosteal osteoma is very rare ● Peak incidence: 30–50 years of age ● No sex predilection.

▶ **Etiology, pathophysiology, pathogenesis**
Benign lesion ● Composed of well-differentiated mature bone tissue ● Predominantly lamellar structure ● Very slow growth.
Classification:
– Classic osteoma (ivory exostosis, ivory osteoma): external table of calvaria, frontal sinus, ethmoidal cells.
– Juxtacortical (parosteal) osteoma: long bones (especially femur), grows on the outer surface of the bone.
– Osteoma medullare (endosteoma, island of compact bone, bone island): only in spongy bone, presents as an island of dense, compact bone.

Imaging Signs
....

▶ **Modality of choice**
Radiography ● If diagnosis uncertain (parosteal location), CT to distinguish from mature myositis ossificans.

▶ **Radiographic findings**
Ivory-like mass ● Located on bone surface (or in medullary space) ● Round or oval-shaped ● Smooth borders ● Well-demarcated and homogeneously sclerotic lesion ● No space between lesion and cortex.

▶ **CT findings**
Distinguish parosteal osteoma from myositis ossificans ● Myositis ossificans characterized by a zonal pattern with a radiolucent central area of immature bone tissue surrounded by a dense peripheral zone (ring) of mature bone.

▶ **MRI findings**
Usually an incidental finding ● Hypointense on T1-weighted and T2-weighted images ● Possibly a small amount of perilesional edema (not considered a criterion of malignancy if lesion is smaller than 3 cm and has an otherwise typical appearance).

▶ **Nuclear medicine**
Typical: negative (lesion is inactive) ● Atypical: positive (active growth).

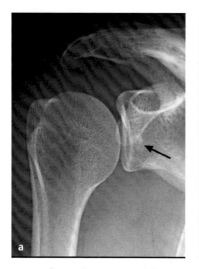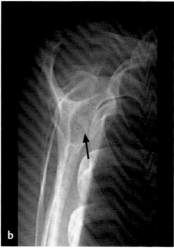

Fig. 1.1 a, b Small osteoma medullare in the glenoid cavity. Most osteomas are readily diagnosed on radiographs.
a AP view. The well-defined sclerotic bone island (arrow) is partly obscured.
b Outlet view radiograph. The sclerotic bone island is easily recognized. Angulated acromion.

Clinical Aspects

▶ **Typical presentation**
  Usually asymptomatic ● Incidental finding on imaging studies ● Osteomas of the paranasal sinuses can obstruct the ostia, blocking drainage and causing headache.
▶ **Treatment options**
  Surgical excision of symptomatic lesions.
▶ **Course and prognosis**
  No risk of recurrence after removal.
▶ **What does the clinician want to know?**
  Differential diagnosis to distinguish from other conditions (see below).

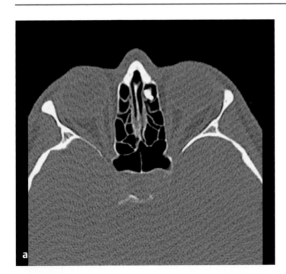

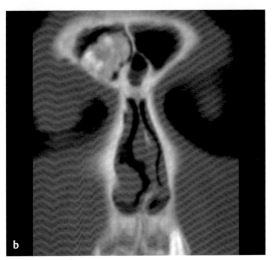

Fig. 1.2 a, b Osteoma of the skull. CT. **a** Small, exophytic osteoma involving the anterior ethmoidal cells. **b** Larger osteoma of the frontal sinus. The typically sessile lesion, located on the wall of the sinus, is sharply marginated and has a homogeneously sclerotic appearance.

Tumors

Differential Diagnosis

Osteochondroma	– Lesion is continuous with host bone cortex
Juxtacortical myositis ossificans	– Zonal pattern: peripheral zone of mature bone
Parosteal osteosarcoma	– Less opaque and homogeneous radiographic appearance
Periosteal osteoblastoma	– Round/oval-shaped, sessile lesion located on the cortex – Radiopacity varies
Ossifying parosteal lipoma	– Lobulated mass – Contains irregular foci of ossification and radiolucent adipose tissue
Melorheostosis	– Cortical expansion resembling dripping candle wax – Longer extent
Meningioma	– Dural tail sign on MRI
Sclerotic metastasis	– More rapid growth – Margins may be indistinct – Negative bone and PET scans are strongly suggestive of osteoma rather than (active) metastasis

Tips and Pitfalls

Mistaking the lesion for a metastasis.

Selected References

Greenspan A. Skelettradiologie. 3rd ed. Munich: Urban & Fischer, 2003: 633–637

White LM, Kandel R. Osteoid-producing tumors of bone. Semin Musculoskelet Radiol 2000 4(1): 25–43

Leone A, Costantini A, Guglielmi G, Settecasi C, Priolo F. Primary bone tumors and pseudo-tumors of the lumbosacral spine. Rays 2000; 25(1): 89–103

Greenspan A. Bone island (enostosis): current concept—a review. Skeletal Radiol 1995; 24(2): 111–115

Definition

▶ **Epidemiology**
4–11% of all benign bone tumors • Usually diagnosed during adolescence • Affects men twice as often as women • Generally found in diaphyseal or metaphyseal/diaphyseal region in long bones (65%), in phalanges (20%), or in spine (10%) • Cortical, medullary, or periosteal location; intracapsular lesions may occur in the hip • Multicentric or multifocal osteoid osteomas are very rare.

▶ **Etiology, pathophysiology, pathogenesis**
Smallish (< 1 cm) osteoblastic, painful tumor • High degree of osteoid formation • Highly vascular central nidus (if calcified, "mature" osteoid osteoma) • Surrounding reactive new bone formation • Nidus histology: loose, highly vascularized connective tissue with irregular strands of trabecular bone and highly proliferative, active osteoblasts without atypia • Classified by location:
  – Cortical (80%).
  – Intra-articular or juxta-articular (mostly femoral neck, hands, feet, and spine).
  – Subperiosteal (mostly femoral neck, hands, and feet, especially talar neck).

Imaging Signs

▶ **Modality of choice**
Radiography • Nuclear medicine • CT • MRI.

▶ **Radiographic findings**
Osteolytic area (nidus) about the size of a grain of rice located on the cortex with surrounding sclerosis • Often considerable cortical thickening • Sclerosis may be absent in intra-articular osteoid osteoma • Joint effusion • Abnormal alignment seen in the case of vertebral lesions.

▶ **CT findings**
Better depiction of nidus with varying degrees of mineralization (absent, punctate, ring-shaped, or, rarely, uniform) • Early nidus enhancement after administration of contrast material • Surrounding sclerosis.

▶ **MRI findings**
On T1-weighted images nidus is isointense to muscle, slightly hyperintense on T2-weighted images • Fat-saturated T1-weighted sequences depict enhancement after contrast administration especially well • On fat-saturated T2-weighted turbo spin-echo (TSE) or short-inversion-time inversion recovery (STIR) sequences extensive marrow edema is characteristic • This may be a sign of osteoid osteoma if consistent with symptom constellation (e.g., younger patient, spontaneous pain mostly at night, no trauma) • A targeted search for the nidus should be made (on CT if necessary) • Intra-articular osteoid osteoma often accompanied by synovitis and joint effusion.

▶ **Nuclear medicine**
Characteristic "double-density" sign: highly active central area surrounded by less active zone of lower levels of tracer uptake.

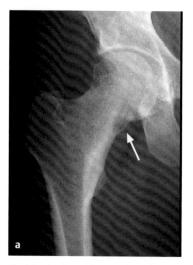
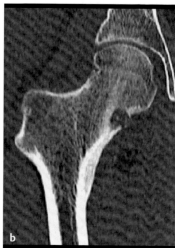

Fig. 1.3 a, b   Osteoid osteoma at the concavity of the femoral neck, its base on the cortex. The patient had typical clinical symptoms of night pain relieved by aspirin.
a Radiograph. 8-mm osteolytic lesion with erosion of the cortex (arrow).
b CT, coronal reconstruction. Small calcifications within the nidus.

Clinical Aspects

▶ **Typical presentation**
Diffuse night pain that cannot be precisely localized • Pain responds well to salicylates • Spinal lesions associated with painful alignment abnormalities (scoliosis, kyphoscoliosis, lordosis, torticollis) • In alignment abnormalities, curvature is concave toward the lesion • Symptoms of intra-articular osteoid osteoma resemble arthritis or osteoarthritis.

▶ **Treatment options**
Curettage of the nidus • CT-guided radiofrequency ablation • Alternatively, drill excision or ablation with ethanol.

▶ **Course and prognosis**
Possible spontaneous regression • Stimulation of the growth plate in skeletally immature patients may lead to hypertrophy of the affected extremity or scoliosis, which can be reversible with early therapy.

▶ **What does the clinician want to know?**
Size • Location • Distinguish from stress fracture or inflammation.

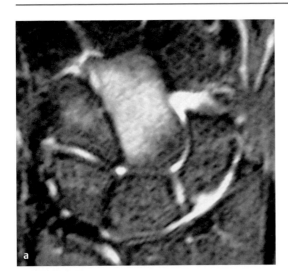

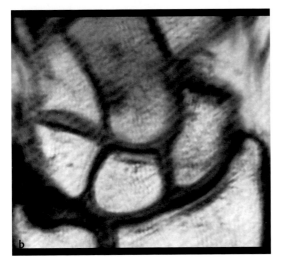

Fig. 1.4 a, b
Osteoid osteoma in the capitate. Long-standing history (many years) of pain without definite diagnosis.
a MRI, STIR sequence. Marked edema involving nearly the entire bone.
b Hypointense nidus on a T1-weighted sequence.

Differential Diagnosis

Stress fracture	– Fracture line and surrounding reaction usually run perpendicular to cortex
	– Symptoms on weight-bearing
	– Virtually no response to salicylates
	– History and location
Sclerosing osteoperiostitis	– Thickening purely periosteal
	– No cortical thickening toward the marrow
Osteomyelitis, Brodie abscess	– Abscess cavity, sequestra, cloacae, sinus tract
	– Usually larger with confluent areas
Bone infarct	– Serpiginous marginal sclerosis
	– Usually larger than 1 cm
	– Osteonecrosis usually subarticular
	– Smaller amount of edema relative to lesion size
Osteoma	– No nidus, no surrounding reaction

Tips and Pitfalls

Mistaking the lesion for a stress fracture or osteomyelitis.

Selected References

Allen SD, Saifuddin A. Imaging of intra-articular osteoid osteoma. Clin Radiol 2003; 58(11): 845–852

Woertler K. Benign bone tumors and tumor-like lesions: value of cross-sectional imaging. Eur Radiol 2003; 13(8): 1820–1835

Definition

▶ **Epidemiology**
Benign intraosseous tumor composed of well-differentiated cartilaginous tissue • Most common tumor affecting small tubular bones of the hand and foot (more than 60% in the middle and distal thirds of the metacarpals or metatarsals and proximal third of the phalanges) • Also affects long tubular bones (proximal femur, proximal humerus) and pelvis • Usually diaphyseal, rarely metaphyseal • Multiple lesions possible (Ollier disease or enchondromatosis, Maffucci syndrome) with malignant transformation (20%) • Manifestation usually between 20 and 40 years of age • No sex predilection.

▶ **Etiology, pathophysiology, pathogenesis**
Presumably arises from well-differentiated cartilaginous tissue that is displaced from the growth plate during development • Relatively small tumors with slow growth • Histology varies by location • Lesions in the long tubular bones and axial skeleton are usually lobulated and made up of hyaline cartilage with low cellularity • Enchondromas occurring in small tubular bones are more cellular, but without increased risk of malignant transformation.

Imaging Signs

▶ **Modality of choice**
Radiography • CT • MRI (only when diagnosis is uncertain and treatment is warranted).

▶ **Radiographic findings**
Radiographs in two planes (AP and lateral) • Relatively sharply defined bone destruction without significant marginal sclerosis • Typical dot-like, fluffy, popcorn-like calcifications within the lesion, especially in the small tubular bones of the hand and foot • May be more difficult to visualize in the long bones • Possible expansile growth • Slight cortical erosions ("scalloping") may be present, but are not a certain sign of malignant transformation • Malignant transformation should be suspected when there is cortical breakthrough, rapid growth with purely lytic areas adjacent to calcifying regions, and expansion into the soft tissue • Interpretation in conjunction with clinical presentation.
Ollier disease: Multiple enchondromas • Lesions often larger • Unilateral distribution.
Maffucci syndrome: Multiple enchondromas with concomitant soft-tissue hemangiomas • Often calcifications.

▶ **CT findings**
Sharply demarcated area of bone destruction without significant marginal sclerosis • Fluffy calcifications within the tumor • Possible pathologic fracture • During the course of disease, cortical thinning by more than two-thirds may imply malignant transformation • Expansion into adjacent soft tissues may be seen.

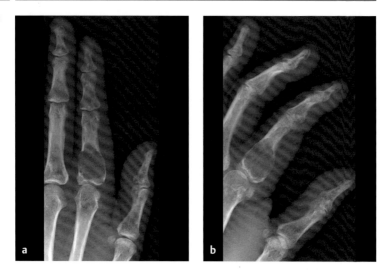

Fig. 1.5 a, b Enchondroma in proximal phalanx of the index finger. Radiograph showing extensive, sharply-defined bone lesion with slight cortical thinning and tiny matrix calcifications. Incidental finding of multiple, small sclerotic islands (osteopoikilosis).

▶ **MRI findings**
Often an incidental finding ● Characteristic signal of cartilage with high signal intensity on T2-weighted and PD-weighted images ● Intermediate signal intensity on T1-weighted images ● Fluffy calcifications appearing as foci with markedly decreased signal intensity ● Readily distinguishable from bone infarct by characteristic lobular morphology and dot-like calcifications ● Expansion into adjacent soft tissues may be seen.

▶ **Nuclear medicine**
Usually no increase in activity ● Slightly increased activity in actively calcifying lesions, but notably less intense than in chondrosarcoma.

Clinical Aspects

▶ **Typical presentation**
Frequently asymptomatic ● No pain ● Enlarged phalanx of the affected hand possible ● At other locations, usually an incidental finding ● Occasionally, pathologic fracture ● New pain related to the lesion may indicate malignant transformation.

▶ **Treatment options**

Asymptomatic lesions do not require treatment ● Troublesome enchondromas of the hand may be treated with curettage and spongiosaplasty ● Rarely, resection and amputation are necessary.

▶ **Course and prognosis**

Risk of malignant transformation is greater in enchondroma than in osteochondroma, but less than in enchondromatosis ● Risk is especially high in large lesions closer to the trunk, enchondromas expanding into the soft tissues, and lesions growing after closure of the growth plate.

▶ **What does the clinician want to know?**

Extent of the lesion ● Fracture risk ● Features indicative of malignant transformation (chondrosarcoma) ● Distinction from other bone tumors.

Differential Diagnosis

Bone infarct	– Typically peripheral, garland-like sclerosis
	– No comma-shaped, dotted calcifications
	– No bone expansion

Tips and Pitfalls

Mistaking the lesion for a malignant bone tumor or bone infarct.

Selected References

Wang K, Allen L, Fung E, Chan CC, Chan JC, Griffith JF. Bone scintigraphy in common tumors with osteolytic components. Clin Nucl Med 2005; 30(10): 655–671

Woertler K. Benign bone tumors and tumor-like lesions: value of cross-sectional imaging. Eur Radiol 2003; 13(8): 1820–1835

Schaser KD, Bail HJ, Haas NP, Melcher I. Treatment concepts of benign bone tumors and tumor-like bone lesions. Chirurg 2002; 73(12): 1181–1190

Erlemann R. Benign cartilaginous tumors. Radiologe 2001; 41(7): 548–559

Flemming DJ, Murphey MD. Enchondroma and chondrosarcoma. Semin Musculoskelet Radiol 2000; 4(1): 59–71

Brien EW, Mirra JM, Kerr R. Benign and malignant cartilage tumors of bone and joint: their anatomic and theoretical basis with an emphasis on radiology, pathology and clinical biology. I. The intramedullary cartilage tumors. Skeletal Radiol 1997; 26(6): 325–353

1 Osteochondroma (Cartilaginous Exostosis)

Definition

▶ **Epidemiology**
Most common benign bone tumor ● Often an incidental finding ● 20–50% of all benign bone tumors ● 10–15% of all bone tumors ● Manifestation in the first 2 decades of life ● No sex predilection.

▶ **Etiology, pathophysiology, pathogenesis**
Benign bone and cartilage-producing tumor ● Bony protuberance covered by hyaline cartilage ● Grows during childhood with enchondral ossification of the cartilage cap ● Growth of the lesion ceases when skeletal maturity is reached.
Multiple cartilaginous exostoses: Special variant of osteochondroma ● Autosomal dominant inheritance ● Multiple osteochondromas ● Increased risk of malignant transformation (10–20%).

Imaging Signs

▶ **Modality of choice**
Radiographs in two planes.

▶ **Pathognomonic findings**
Cauliflower-like bony outgrowth that is continuous with underlying cortical and spongy bone.

▶ **Radiographic findings**
Stalked or sessile osteochondroma ● Lesion grows outwardly, is continuous with underlying spongy and cortical bone, and has a broad-based, conical, or cauliflower-like appearance ● Has a trabecular matrix ● Smooth, clearly defined borders ● May be bizarrely configured ● Location close to the metaphysis or diaphyseal/metaphyseal on long tubular bones (especially femur, tibia, humerus) ● Cartilage cap is usually not visible on radiographs, but may demonstrate patchy calcifications.

▶ **MRI findings**
Osteochondroma evidenced by continuity between isointense signal in the lesion and the tubular bone ● MRI is the modality of choice for determining cartilage cap thickness ● Markedly hyperintense cartilage cap on T2-weighted spin-echo (SE) or fat-saturated images (thickness greater than 2 cm suggests malignancy!).

Clinical Aspects

▶ **Typical presentation**
Smaller exostoses often remain undetected or are discovered as incidental findings ● Larger cartilaginous exostoses may impinge on adjacent joints or nerves and vessels.

▶ **Treatment options**
Resection only in patients with symptoms arising from mechanical factors or with suspected malignancy.

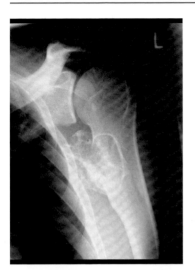

Fig. 1.6 Osteochondroma. AP radiograph of the left humerus in a 23-year-old man with a typical cauliflower-like osteochondroma on the proximal humerus.

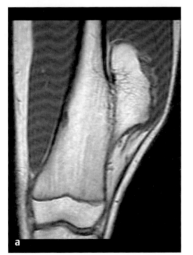

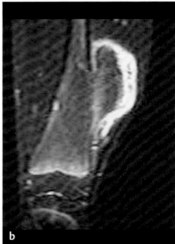

Fig. 1.7 Osteochondroma. A 12-year-old girl with a large cartilaginous exostosis on the distal femoral shaft. MRI. Signal intensity similar to fat on T1-weighted SE images (**a**). Markedly hyperintense cartilage cap discernible on fat-saturated STIR images (**b**) measuring 1.5 cm at its greatest thickness. The exostosis was removed. No malignancy was found.

▶ **Course and prognosis**
Spontaneous regression ● Lesion stops growing after puberty ends ● Risk of malignant transformation is less than 1% ● Malignant degeneration should be suspected if there is renewed growth of the lesion or pain after cessation of growth ● Possible bursa formation on the cartilage cap mimicking growth of the lesion.

▶ **What does the clinician want to know?**
Location ● Signs of malignant transformation ● Thickness of cartilage cap.

Differential Diagnosis
. . . .

Chondrosarcoma	– Indistinct border
	– Pain
	– Sudden growth in size
	– Cartilage cap thicker than 2 cm

Tips and Pitfalls
. . . .

Mistaking the lesion for a malignant bone tumor.

Selected References

Brien EW, Mirra JM, Luck JV Jr. Benign and malignant cartilage tumors of bone and joint: their anatomic and theoretical basis with an emphasis on radiology, pathology and clinical biology. II. Juxtacortical cartilage tumors. Skeletal Radiol 1999; 28(1): 1–20

Murphey MD, Choi JJ, Kransdorf MJ, Flemming DJ, Gannon FH. Imaging of osteochondroma: variants and complications with radiologic-pathologic correlation. Radiographics 2000; 20(5): 1407–1434

Definition

▶ **Epidemiology**
First and second decades of life ● More common in boys than girls.

▶ **Etiology, pathophysiology, pathogenesis**
Classic "tumor-like" lesion ● Developmental defect in the metaphysis of long bones ● 90% in the legs (especially tibia) ● Defect filled with fibrous connective tissue connected to overlying periosteum ● Fibrous cortical defects that are purely cortical or involve the medullary space are termed nonossifying fibromas (NOF) ● Increased incidence in patients with neurofibromatosis.

Imaging Signs

▶ **Modality of choice**
Radiographs in two planes.

▶ **Pathognomonic findings**
Grape-like lucency with sclerotic rim ● Usually affects distal tibia.

▶ **Radiographic findings**
Sharply defined multilocular radiolucent zone ● Surrounding sclerotic rim ● Long tubular bones (especially lower extremity) ● Metadiaphyseal ● Eccentric, cortical lesion ● Healing with full recovery or complete sclerosis of the lesion.

▶ **MRI findings**
Hypointense on T1-weighted SE images ● Hypointense to surrounding fatty marrow on T2-weighted TSE images.

Clinical Aspects

▶ **Typical presentation**
Asymptomatic ● Frequently an incidental finding on radiographs ● Spontaneous fracture very rare.

▶ **Treatment options**
No treatment needed.

▶ **Course and prognosis**
Heals spontaneously ● No malignant degeneration.

▶ **What does the clinician want to know?**
Definitive diagnosis.

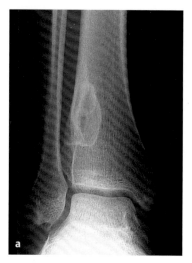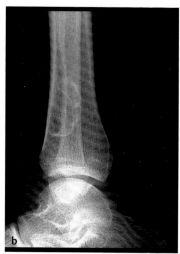

Fig. 1.8 a, b Nonossifying fibroma (NOF). Radiograph of the ankle joint shown in two planes in a 17-year-old boy. Multilocular radiolucency with peripheral sclerosis in the distal tibia.

Fig. 1.9 A 28-year-old woman with a resolved NOF lesion on the distal tibia. Circumscribed sclerotic zone at a typical site.

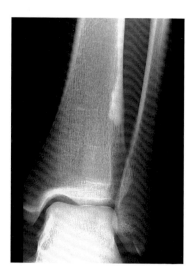

Differential Diagnosis

Juvenile or aneurysmal bone cyst	– Epiphyseal/metaphyseal expansile cystic lesion – Fluid detection on MRI
Osteomyelitis	– Osseous destruction with indistinct borders – Periosteal reaction
Fibrous dysplasia	– "Ground-glass" opacity – Usually fairly wide sclerotic rim

Tips and Pitfalls

Include differential diagnoses in the radiology report. Radiological findings are unambiguously diagnostic for NOF. NOFs are regarded as "leave-me-alone lesions" and no further investigations, including biopsy, are indicated.

Selected References

Goodin GS, Shulkin BL, Kaufman RA, McCarville MB. PET/CT characterization of fibro-osseous defects in children: 18F-FDG uptake can mimic metastatic disease. AJR Am J Roentgenol 2006; 187: 1124–1128

Yaw KM. Pediatric bone tumors [review]. Semin Surg Oncol 1999; 16(2): 173–183

Definition

▶ **Epidemiology**
Most common tumor-like lesion • Age of manifestation: 1st and 2nd decades.

▶ **Etiology, pathophysiology, pathogenesis**
Etiology unclear • Spongy bone and bone marrow are replaced by fibro-osseous tissue with secondary remodeling and formation of woven bone.
– Monostotic: affects 70–80% with predilection for long bones.
– Polyostotic: affects 20–30% with bilateral involvement and predilection for one side.
– Albright syndrome: triad of polyostotic fibrous dysplasia, café-au-lait spots, and precocious puberty.

Imaging Signs

▶ **Modality of choice**
Conventional radiographs • CT or MRI if differential diagnosis is difficult.

▶ **Pathognomonic findings**
Geographic, round, lytic, ground-glass appearance • Metadiaphyseal location • Surrounding sclerotic rim.

▶ **Radiographic findings**
Most common locations: metadiaphyseal region of humerus or femur, pelvis, ribs, cranium • Smoothly bordered lucencies with or without cortical thinning and expansion, Lodwick I lesion • Loss of structure of spongy bone • Narrow transitional zone • Usually sclerotic rim • Ground-glass appearance (corresponding to immature osteoid) and "soap-bubble" appearance are typical • Cranial lesions: pagetoid, sclerotic, cystoid forms • Bowing of long tubular bones is possible (shepherd's crook deformity) • Honeycomb appearance common on flat bones.

▶ **CT findings**
CT can often better depict ground-glass opacity.

▶ **MRI findings**
Soft-tissue-intensity, sharply defined areas that are hypointense on T1-weighted SE images • Hypointense on T2-weighted TSE images • Moderately hyperintense on fat-saturated images (e.g., STIR) • Homogeneously enhancing • Predominantly homogeneous signal intensity • Lesions with cystic transformation and hemorrhage may have inhomogeneous signal intensity with signal intensity equal to that of fluid.

▶ **Nuclear medicine**
Tracer accumulation depends on degree of vascularization and new bone formation.

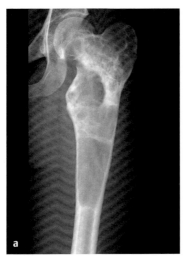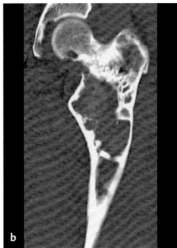

Fig. 1.10 a, b   A 27-year-old woman with fibrous dysplasia affecting the proximal femur.
a Plain radiograph showing soap-bubble appearance in the femur with typical ground-glass opacity corresponding to immature osteoid. Typical shepherd's crook deformity.
b Coronal reconstruction of MSCT views.

Clinical Aspects

▶ **Typical presentation**
   Bone pain ● Frequently an incidental clinical finding ● Pathologic fractures are rare.

▶ **Treatment options**
   Stabilization of bones at risk of fracture ● No other therapy needed.

▶ **Course and prognosis**
   Growth tends to cease with puberty ● Disease occasionally becomes active again during pregnancy or with estrogen therapy ● Malignant degeneration is uncommon (< 0.5 %).

▶ **What does the clinician want to know?**
   Size of lesion ● Cortical thinning ● Fracture.

Fig. 1.11 a–d
Fibrous dysplasia.
A 48-year-old woman with fibrous dysplasia affecting the distal humerus.
a Radiograph showing geographic lesion with cystic expansion of the humeral shaft. Typical ground-glass appearance.
b Axial T1-weighted SE sequence. Hypointense lesion and cortical thinning.

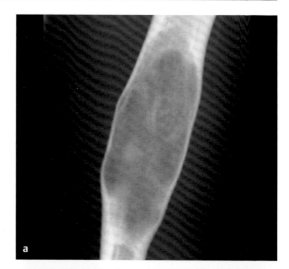

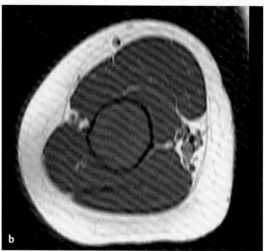

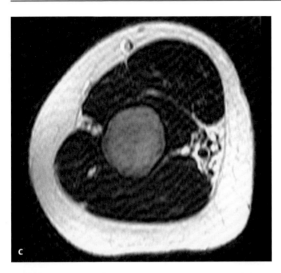

c T2-weighted TSE sequence. Hypointense signal relative to normal fatty marrow.

d T1-weighted SE sequence after administration of Gd-DTPA. Homogeneous enhancement of the lesion.

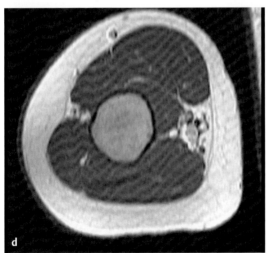

Differential Diagnosis

Juvenile bone cyst	– No ground-glass opacity on radiographs – MRI reveals cystic lesion with only peripheral enhancement after contrast administration
NOF	– No ground-glass opacity – Grows from cortical bone – Eccentrically located
Aneurysmal bone cyst	– No ground-glass opacity – Cystic on MRI
Eosinophilic granuloma	– No ground-glass opacity (CT)

Tips and Pitfalls

Mistaking the lesion for a malignant bone tumor ● Biopsy only in exceptional circumstances ● "Leave-me-alone" lesion.

Selected References

Fitzpatrick KA, Taljanovic MS, Speer DP et al. Imaging findings of fibrous dysplasia with histopathologic and intraoperative correlation. AJR Am J Roentgenol 2004; 182(6): 1389–1398

Ritschel P, Karnel F, Hajek P. Fibrous metaphyseal defects: determination of their origin and natural history using a radiomorphological study. Skeletal Radiol 1988; 17(1): 8–15

Bertoni F, Fernando Arias L, Alberghini M, Bacchini P. Fibrous dysplasia with degenerative atypia: a benign lesion potentially mistaken for sarcoma. Arch Pathol Lab Med 2004; 128(7): 794–796

Kyriakos M, McDonald D, Sundaram M. Fibrous dysplasia with cartilaginous differentiation ("fibrocartilaginous dysplasia"): a review, with an illustrative case followed for 18 years. Skeletal Radiol 2004; 33(1): 51–62

Shah ZK, Peh WC, Koh WL, Shek TW. Magnetic resonance imaging appearances of fibrous dysplasia. Br J Radiol 2005; 78(936): 1104–1115

Definition

▶ **Epidemiology**
First and second decades of life ● Peak incidence around age 13 ● 6% of all benign osseous bone lesions ● Affects boys twice as often as girls.

▶ **Etiology, pathophysiology, pathogenesis**
Unknown etiology ● Unicameral bone cyst ● Filled with serous, yellowish fluid ● Cyst wall composed of well-vascularized trabecular network ● Lined by well-vascularized connective-tissue membrane.

Imaging Signs

▶ **Modality of choice**
Radiographs in two planes ● MRI if differential diagnosis is uncertain.

▶ **Radiographic findings**
Almost exclusively metaphyseal or metadiaphyseal (less frequently diaphyseal) regions of long tubular bones, especially proximal humerus (50%) and femur (25%) ● Rarely affects pelvis, calcaneus, tibia, or fibula ● Centrally located, sharply bordered, geographic lesion (may contain "pseudotrabeculae") ● Often sclerotic rim ● Expansion of bone uncommon ● If expansion present, possible thin periosteal shell ● Intralesional fragment within the cyst after pathologic fracture ("fallen fragment" sign) is pathognomonic but rare.

▶ **CT findings**
As radiographic findings ● Distinguish between unicameral and multilocular cyst ● Pathologic fracture.

▶ **MRI findings**
Signal intensity equal to that of fluid ● Markedly hyperintense on T2-weighted SE images ● Hypointense on T1-weighted SE images ● No intralesional contrast enhancement ● Enhancement of cyst margin possible ● If hemorrhage present, hyperintense signal on T1-weighted SE and fat-saturated T1-weighted images ● Fluid–fluid levels possible.

Clinical Aspects

▶ **Typical presentation**
Usually asymptomatic ● Often manifests with pathologic fracture after trivial trauma.

▶ **Treatment options**
Often heals spontaneously ● Hence conservative treatment ● Treatment options include cortisone injections, curettage, and spongiosaplasty.

▶ **Course and prognosis**
Good prognosis ● High rate of spontaneous healing ● Healing within 6–12 months after steroid injection.

▶ **What does the clinician want to know?**
Location and size of lesion ● Stability ● Pathologic fracture.

Fig. 1.12 Juvenile bone cyst. AP femoral radiograph in a 27-year-old woman with a juvenile bone cyst in the left femoral neck. Typical benign, sharply defined, geographic lesion.

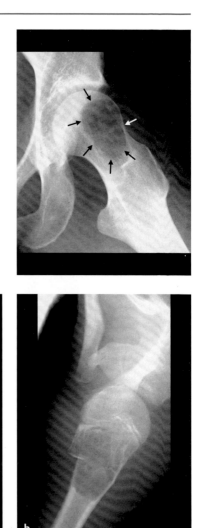

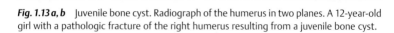

Fig. 1.13 a, b Juvenile bone cyst. Radiograph of the humerus in two planes. A 12-year-old girl with a pathologic fracture of the right humerus resulting from a juvenile bone cyst.

Differential Diagnosis

Aneurysmal bone cyst	– Differential diagnosis—even histological—is difficult if lesion is expansile – Location more eccentric – Growth more expansile – MRI demonstrates well-vascularized septa
Giant cell tumor	– Epiphyseal location – Borders generally slightly less distinct – MRI shows solid formations that enhance after contrast administration
Fibrous dysplasia	– Radiography: sclerotic margin, ground-glass opacity – MRI shows solid tissue that enhances after contrast administration, soft-tissue density
Calcaneal lipoma	– Centrally located, punctate calcification – Mimics fat on CT and MRI studies

Tips and Pitfalls

Mistaking the lesion for a malignant bone tumor.

Selected References

Bancroft LW, Peterson JJ, Kransdorf MJ. Cysts, geodes, and erosions. Radiol Clin North Am 2004; 42(1): 73–87

Definition
....

▶ **Epidemiology**
Predominantly affects children and adolescents (90% of patients are under age 20).

▶ **Etiology, pathophysiology, pathogenesis**
Blood-filled cavities containing connective tissue septa ● Contains trabeculae or osteoid tissue and osteoclastic giant cells ● Lesions are primary or secondary, arising after cystic degeneration of pre-existing lesions (e.g., benign or malignant bone tumors) or trauma.

Imaging Signs
....

▶ **Modality of choice**
Conventional radiography ● MRI.

▶ **Pathognomonic findings**
Eccentric cystic bone lesion at a metaphyseal location ● Cortical expansion.

▶ **Radiographic findings**
Usually large, eccentric lesion in the metaphyseal region ● Well-defined margin ● No or minimal sclerosis ● Often septated ● Possible expansion into the soft tissues ● Endosteal scalloping.

▶ **MRI findings**
Hypointense on T1-weighted SE images ● Markedly hyperintense on T2-weighted SE images (signal intensity equal to that of fluid) ● Signal intensity may be heterogeneous in parts ● Fluid–fluid levels (sedimentation of corpuscular components of blood) are typical but not pathognomonic ● Nonenhancing or only peripherally enhancing after contrast administration ● Periphery of the lesion may contain solid components ● Paraosseous soft-tissue component may be present.

Clinical Aspects
....

▶ **Typical presentation**
Nonspecific ● Pain ● Swelling.

▶ **Treatment options**
Curettage and cancellous bone graft ● Alternatively, surgical excision of entire lesion ● Recurrence rate: 20–40%.

▶ **Course and prognosis**
Potential for rapid growth leading to pathologic fracture.

▶ **What does the clinician want to know?**
Extent ● Signs of malignancy ● Distinguish from other bone tumors.

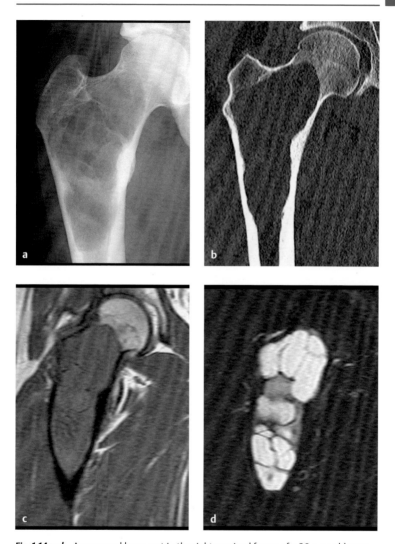

Fig. 1.14 a–d Aneurysmal bone cyst in the right proximal femur of a 26-year-old man.
a AP radiograph showing geographic, well-defined, osteolytic lesion in the right proximal femur.
b CT (coronal reconstruction) showing bone lysis with endosteal scalloping.
c MRI, T1-weighted SE/T1-weighted sequence. The tumor is hypointense to normal fatty marrow.
d MRI, STIR sequence. Signal intensity and septation are typical of aneurysmal bone cyst.

Tumors

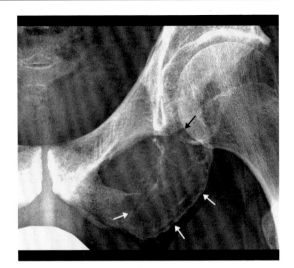

Fig. 1.15 AP radiograph of left ischium in a 45-year-old man showing aneurysmal bone cyst in the left ischium. Ischium shows bone lysis and a "bubbly" appearance.

Differential Diagnosis

Simple bone cyst	– Frequently indistinguishable on radiographs
	– May also exhibit fluid–fluid levels, but never "solid", enhancing structures
Giant cell tumor	– Epiphyseal location
	– MRI: solid, homogeneously enhancing tumor
Nonossifying fibroma	– Marked sclerotic rim
	– Eccentrically located cortical lesion
	– No typical cystic signal on MRI studies (hypointense on T1-weighted SE images, hypointense on T2-weighted TSE images, slightly hyperintense on STIR images)

Tips and Pitfalls

Mistaking the lesion for a metastasis or malignant bone tumor.

Selected References

Kransdorf MJ, Sweet DE. Aneurysmal bone cyst: concept, controversy, clinical presentation, and imaging. AJR Am J Roentgenol 1995; 164(3): 573–580

Mendenhall WM, Zlotecki RA, Gibbs CP, Reith JD, Scarborough MT, Mendenhall NP. Aneurysmal bone cyst. Am J Clin Oncol 2006; 29(3): 311–315

Maiya S, Davies M, Evans N, Grimer J. Surface aneurysmal bone cysts: a pictorial review. Eur Radiol 2002; 12(1): 99–108

Asaumi J, Konouchi H, Hisatomi M, et al. MR features of aneurysmal bone cyst of the mandible and characteristics distinguishing it from other lesions. Eur J Radiol 2003; 45(2): 108–112

Definition

▶ **Epidemiology**
10% of all bone tumors • 20% of all benign bone tumors • Age predilection: 20–40 years • Peak incidence in 3rd decade of life • No sex predilection.

▶ **Etiology, pathophysiology, pathogenesis**
Etiology unclear • Aggressively growing, usually benign tumor • Highly vascular tissue • Mononuclear spindle cells and giant cells within the tumor (giant cells are also present in other lesions such as aneurysmal bone cysts) • Three grades are distinguished: benign (I), semi-malignant (II), and malignant (III) • Aneurysmal bone cysts may be found in a giant cell tumor • Secondary giant cell tumors are occasionally seen in Paget disease (patients over 60 years of age).

Imaging Signs

▶ **Modality of choice**
Radiography.

▶ **Pathognomonic findings**
Well-demarcated osteolytic lesion in the epiphyseal/metaphyseal region.

▶ **Radiographic/CT findings**
Eccentric location • Relatively well-defined osteolytic lesion (Lodwick IB–C) • Rapidly growing lesions may have indistinct margins • Internal septation in 50% • Residual trabeculae imply less aggressive growth • Often cortical erosion • Usually no sclerotic rim, no matrix calcification, and no periosteal reaction • Occasional soft-tissue component, which may be bordered in part by a thin shell of bone (neocortex) • Potential for aggressive growth (Lodwick II) • Typical location: epiphyseal/metaphyseal, rarely metadiaphyseal • Predilection for the knee, distal radius, and spine (usually partly in the posterior portion of the vertebral body and in the vertebral arch).

▶ **MRI findings**
Soft-tissue density • Hypointense on T1-weighted SE images • Hyperintense on T2-weighted SE images (although no fluid signal) • Usually homogeneous enhancement after contrast administration • Occasional areas of hemorrhage.

▶ **Nuclear medicine**
High levels of tracer accumulation, but no correlation between the degree of uptake and histology.

Clinical Aspects

▶ **Typical presentation**
Local pain.

▶ **Treatment options**
Primarily surgical: wide resection if possible given location • Subchondral lesions may be treated with curettage and adjuvant therapies (phenol, cryosurgery) as well as defect filling with autologous cancellous bone.

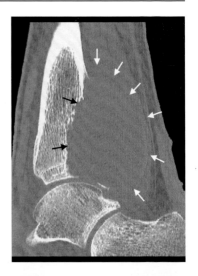

Fig. 1.16 Giant cell tumor. An 8-year-old girl with progressive swelling and pain in the left ankle joint. CT showing well-defined osteolytic lesion on the posterior aspect of the distal tibia. Large, tumorous soft-tissue component.

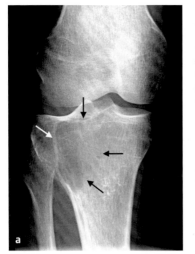
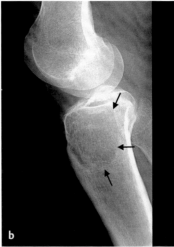

Fig. 1.17 a, b Giant cell tumor. A 38-year-old woman with progressively worsening knee pain. **a** AP and **b** lateral radiographs showing a circumscribed region of bone destruction in the proximal lateral tibial plateau.

▶ **Course and prognosis**
High rate of recurrence (careful attention should be paid to radiographic evidence of recent osteolytic lesions around the primary tumor; diagnosis on MRI) ● Solitary pulmonary metastases occur in 5% and can usually be successfully surgically excised.

▶ **What does the clinician want to know?**
Extent ● Cortical breakthrough ● Soft-tissue infiltration ● Pulmonary metastasis.

Differential Diagnosis

Chondroblastoma	– Chondroid matrix calcifications
	– Usually distinct sclerotic rim
Aneurysmal bone cyst	– Appear very similar on radiographs
	– Location more metaphyseal
	– MRI demonstrates cystic lesion with blood components
	– Usually affects younger patients
Metastasis	– May be difficult to distinguish
	– Usually not at peripheral or epiphyseal location
Juvenile bone cyst	– Sharper borders
	– Metaphyseal location
	– Patient age

Tips and Pitfalls

Confusing the lesion with an aneurysmal bone cyst or malignant bone tumor.

Selected References

Stacy GS, Peabody TD, Dixon LB. Mimics of giant cell tumor of bone. AJR Am J Roentgenol 2003; 181(6): 1583–1589

James SL, Davies AM. Giant cell tumor of bone of the hand and wrist: a review of imaging findings and differential diagnosis. Eur Radiol 2005; 15(9): 1855–1866

Turcotte RE. Giant cell tumor of bone. Orthop Clin North Am 2006; 37(1): 35–51

Lee MJ, Sallomi DF, Munk PL, et al. Giant cell tumours of bone. Clin Radiol 1998; 53(7): 481–489

James SL, Davies AM. Giant-cell tumours of bone of the hand and wrist: a review of imaging findings and differential diagnoses. Eur Radiol 2005; 15(9): 1855–1866

Definition

▶ **Epidemiology**
Can affect patients of any age ● Especially young adults.
▶ **Etiology, pathophysiology, pathogenesis**
Etiology unclear ● Synovial membrane metaplasia ● Nodular cartilage proliferations that may ossify ● Nodular proliferations are attached by stalks to the synovial membrane, which nourishes them ● Primary disease is idiopathic; secondary disease occurs with joint deterioration and arthritis.

Imaging Signs

▶ **Modality of choice**
Radiographs in two planes.
▶ **Radiographic findings**
Round, smoothly bordered calcifications near the joint ● Most common locations: shoulder, elbow, knee ● Often multiple lesions ● Not visible on radiography unless cartilage proliferations become calcified ● MRI or ultrasound studies are thus needed.
▶ **MRI findings**
Multiple, round, low-signal formations in high-signal effusion (T2-weighted).

Clinical Aspects

▶ **Typical presentation**
Pain ● Limited range of motion ● Recurrent joint effusion.
▶ **Treatment options**
Surgical removal.
▶ **Course and prognosis**
If separation from the synovial membrane occurs, there will be intra-articular loose bodies and potential impingement symptoms or reduced mobility ● Joint deterioration is rare.
▶ **What does the clinician want to know?**
Number and location of chondromas ● Degenerative joint changes.

Differential Diagnosis

None ● Appearance is typical.

Selected References

Crotty JM, Monu JU, Pope TL Jr. Synovial osteochondromatosis. Radiol Clin North Am 1996; 34(2): 327–342

Sheldon PJ, Forrester DM, Learch TJ. Imaging of intra-articular masses. Radiographics 2005; 25(1): 105–119

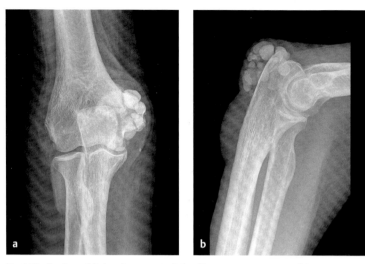

Fig. 1.18 a, b   Synovial chondromatosis of the elbow joint in a 30-year-old man.
a AP and **b** lateral radiographs.

Fig. 1.19 a–d
A 57-year-old pa-
tient with recurrent
effusion in the knee
joint.

a, b Radiographs in
two planes: multi-
ple lesions in the
intercondylar and
posterior portions
of the knee joint.

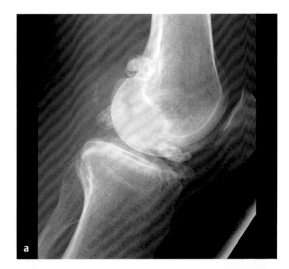

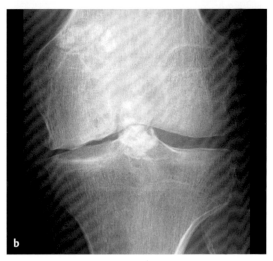

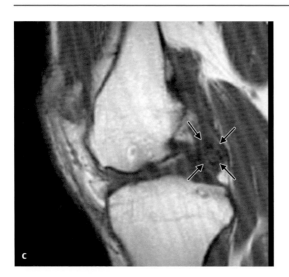

c Sagittal T1-weighted SE sequence. Synovial chondromatosis with hypointense signal.
d Hypointense synovial chondromatosis in the intercondylar region.

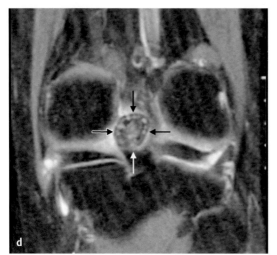

Tumors

Definition

▶ **Epidemiology**

Benign osseous changes arising from newly formed blood vessels ● 2% of all benign and 0.8% of all (benign and malignant) lesions affecting the skeletal system ● Incidence increases with age ● Peak incidence at age 50 ● Women twice as often affected as men ● Usually involves the spine (especially thoracic and lumbar regions) or cranium ● Rarely involves proximal femur ● Typically isolated, although multiple lesions occur in one-third of cases.

▶ **Etiology, pathophysiology, pathogenesis**

Precise etiology uncertain ● Vertebral body hemangiomas possibly arise from local venous stasis corresponding to areas of telangiectasia ● Most bone hemangiomas reside in the medullary cavity, but periosteal or subperiosteal lesions also occur.

Imaging Signs

▶ **Modality of choice**

Conventional radiography ● CT ● MRI ● Angiography.

▶ **Radiographic findings**

Morphology depends on vessel type and location ● Generally trabecular pattern ● Vertebral hemangiomas marked by coarse vertical striations (honeycomb or corduroy appearance) ● Size and shape of vertebral bodies usually maintained ● Cranial hemangiomas are round, osteolytic lesions with a spoke-wheel configuration ● Long, tubular bones demonstrate circumscribed lytic lesions with a spiculated pattern (occasionally also a honeycomb pattern) and marginal sclerosis.

▶ **Angiography**

Variable appearance ● Highly vascular intraosseous processes with hypervascularity ● Corkscrew-like vessels and venous lakes are frequently found ● Other hemangiomas may be completely silent on angiography.

▶ **CT findings**

Punctate pattern on axial slices (polka-dot pattern, cross-sectional appearance of thickened trabeculae) ● Enhancement after intravenous administration of contrast material.

▶ **MRI findings**

Proportion of fat determines signal intensity on T1-weighted images ● Lesions with a low fat content may therefore have an atypical appearance on T1-weighted images, with predominantly low signal intensity ● Hyperintense areas on T2-weighted images correspond to vascular components ● Thickened trabeculae are hypointense on all sequences ● Enhancement after intravenous administration of contrast material.

▶ **Nuclear medicine**

Usually normal, although occasionally a slight increase in activity.

Clinical Aspects

▸ **Typical presentation**

Most vertebral hemangiomas are asymptomatic, incidental findings ● Symptoms arise when the lesion expands epidurally, compressing the nerve roots or spinal cord, or if it leads to pathologic fracture ● Hypervascularity occasionally leads to slight increase in local bone growth.

▸ **Treatment options**

No treatment is needed for asymptomatic hemangiomas ● Symptomatic hemangiomas may be treated with vertebroplasty, embolization, laminectomy, or spondylodesis.

▸ **Course and prognosis**

Good prognosis ● Spontaneous regression possible ● The high risk of hemorrhage associated with surgery may present a challenge in the treatment of symptomatic spinal and pelvic hemangiomas.

▸ **What does the clinician want to know?**

Location and extent of lesion ● Diffuse bone infiltration (angiomatosis).

Differential Diagnosis

Paget disease	– "Picture frame" configuration and increased volume of affected vertebral body – Involvement of adnexa
Multiple myeloma	– Osteolytic lesion – No vertical striations
Metastases	– No fat signal on T1-weighted sequences

Tips and Pitfalls

Mistaking the lesion for a malignancy such as a metastasis or multiple myeloma.

Fig. 1.20 a–d
Vertebral heman-
gioma in T3. CT.
a, b Noncontrast CT
showing lytic lesion.
Distinct and in
places sclerotic bor-
der. Coarse trabecu-
lar architecture with
cord-like and hon-
eycomb appearance
of the lesion.

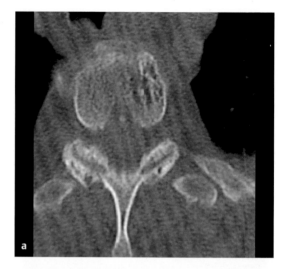

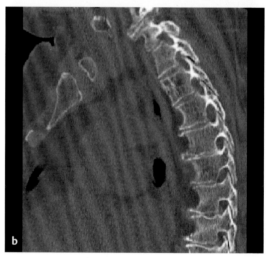

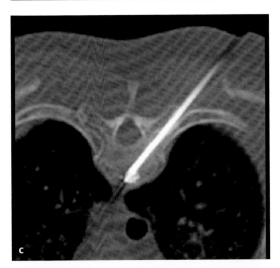

c Vertebroplasty undertaken because of pain. Costotransverse approach from contralateral side.
d Follow-up image after application of bone cement.

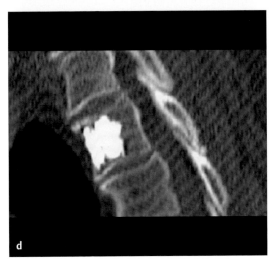

Selected References

Flemming DJ, Murphey MD, Carmichael BB, Bernard SA. Primary tumors of the spine. Semin Musculoskelet Radiol 2000; 4(3): 299–320

Horcajadas AB, Lafuente JL, de la Cruz Burgos R, et al. Ultrasound and MR findings in tumor and tumor-like lesions of the fingers. Eur Radiol 2003; 13(4): 672–685

Mendez JA, Hochmuth A, Boetefuer IC, Schumacher M. Radiologic appearance of a rare primary vertebral lymphangioma. AJNR Am J Neuroradiol 2002; 23(10): 1665–1668

Motamedi K, Ilaslan H, Seeger LL. Imaging of the lumbar spine neoplasms. Semin Ultrasound CT MR 2004; 25(6): 474–489

Porchet F, Sajadi A, Villemure JG. Spinal tumors: clinical aspects, classification and surgical treatment. Schweiz Rundsch Med Prax 2003; 92(45): 1897–1905

Vande Berg BC, Lecouvet FE, Galant C, Maldague BE, Malghem J. Normal variants and frequent marrow alterations that simulate bone marrow lesions at MR imaging. Radiol Clin North Am 2005; 43(4): 761–770

Vilanova JC, Barcelo J, Smirniotopoulos JG, et al. Hemangioma from head to toe: MR imaging with pathologic correlation. Radiographics 2004; 24(2): 367–385

Woertler K. Benign bone tumors and tumor-like lesions: value of cross-sectional imaging. Eur Radiol 2003; 13(8): 1820–1835

Definition

▶ **Epidemiology**
Incidence: 3% of people over age 40 • 90% of patients are over age 40 • Men are affected 1.5–2.1 times as often as women • Predilection for Western Europe, North America, and Australia.

▶ **Etiology, pathophysiology, pathogenesis**
Precise etiology of Paget disease is unknown; debatable whether due to infection of osteoclasts with paramyxoviruses and thus accelerated breakdown of bone tissue and remodeling.

Imaging Signs

▶ **Modality of choice**
Radiography.

▶ **Pathognomonic findings**
Depend on disease stage • Often an increase in bone volume • Sclerotic changes and coarse trabeculations.

▶ **Radiographic findings**
Sites of predilection: pelvis, femur, tibia, cranium, vertebral bodies, sternum • Monostotic and polyostotic forms.
Stages:
 – Stage I (lytic stage): "hot" stage • Increased blood flow • Osteolysis • Lesions in long tubular bones appear as flame-like or wedge-shaped cortical bone destruction.
 – Stage II (mixed stage): mixed osteolytic and sclerotic appearance • Cortical thickening • Coarsening of trabeculae • Enlargement of affected bone.
 – Stage III ("burned-out" stage): sclerosis of bone predominates with possible bone deformities (e.g., saber tibia or shepherd's crook deformity of the femur) • Insufficiency fractures, especially on the convex aspect of the curvature.
Cranium: Calvarial expansion with indistinct borders • Cloudy sclerosis ("cotton wool" appearance on skull radiographs).
Vertebral bodies: Coarse sclerosis of individual vertebrae • Typical findings include increased AP diameter and band-like opacity along the superior and inferior vertebral end plates.

▶ **CT findings**
As radiographic findings • Indicated for clarification of complications (nerve compression, malignant transformation) • Suggestive of malignancy: recent lytic foci in sclerotic bone, soft-tissue component, and paraosseous new bone formation (osteosarcoma) • Differential diagnosis.

▶ **MRI findings**
MRI studies are particularly indicated when there is suspicion of sarcomatous degeneration: recent appearance of hypointense areas on T1-weighted SE images corresponding to hyperintense areas seen in the "burned-out" stage of disease.

Fig. 1.21 A 67-year-old woman with Paget disease affecting the right hemipelvis. Radiographic view of entire pelvis. Burned-out stage of the disease with predominating sclerosis of the right hemipelvis. Lesions typically do not cross the sacroiliac joint. Paget arthropathy of the right hip.

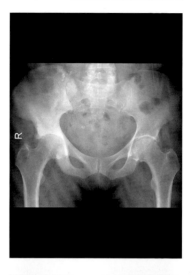

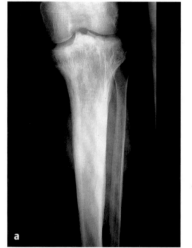

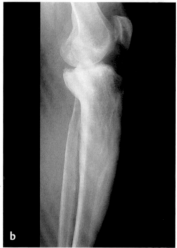

Fig. 1.22 a, b A 72-year-old man with Paget disease of the tibia. **a** AP and **b** lateral tibial radiographs demonstrating bone expansion, sclerosis, and trabecular coarsening.

Stages I–II: Hypointense on T1-weighted SE images • Hyperintense on fat-saturated images, increased enhancement on T1-weighted SE images after administration of contrast material (corresponds to fibrovascular connective tissue) • Indistinguishable from tumor!

Stage III: Signal again isointense to fat • Hyperintense on T1-weighted SE images • Hypointense on fat-saturated images.

▶ **Nuclear medicine**
Areas of increased bone metabolism (hot spots) in stages I and II • Correlates well with disease activity • Confirms or rules out polyostotic form.

Clinical Aspects

▶ **Typical presentation**
Asymptomatic in 90% • Pain is rare; increased local warmth and redness • Alkaline phosphatase levels are typically elevated, while calcium and phosphate levels are normal • New pain related to the lesion suggestive of malignant transformation.

▶ **Treatment options**
Calcitonin (inhibits osteoclastic activity) and bisphosphonates reduce disease activity.

▶ **Course and prognosis**
Follow-up radiographs and serum alkaline phosphatase testing to monitor disease course and activity • Malignant degeneration occurs in 1%: osteosarcoma, fibrosarcoma, giant cell tumor • Occasionally Paget arthropathy develops (joint degeneration and deformity) • Compression of cranial nerves may occur if skull base involved.

▶ **What does the clinician want to know?**
Size and extent of foci of bone remodeling • Pathologic fractures • Bone deformities • Monolocular or multilocular involvement • Signs of malignant transformation.

Differential Diagnosis

Metastasis	– More aggressive growth pattern (Lodwick II–III)
Fibrous dysplasia	– Ground-glass appearance of osteolytic foci
	– Peripheral sclerosis
Vertebral hemangioma	– No enlargement of the vertebra
	– Increased vertical trabeculations

Selected References

Frame B, Marel GM. Paget disease: a review of current knowledge. Radiology 1981; 141(1): 21–24

Sundaram M. Imaging of Paget's disease and fibrous dysplasia of bone. J Bone Miner Res 2006; 21(Suppl 2): P28–30

Definition

▶ **Epidemiology**
Most common bone tumor • Metastatic lesions are usually multiple • Only 10% of bone metastases are solitary lesions.

▶ **Etiology, pathophysiology, pathogenesis**
Hematogenous dissemination of cancer cells to the bone • Osteoclasia and/or osteosclerosis • Most common site: axial skeleton (regions of hematopoietic bone marrow) • Peripheral lesions are rare, usually arising in bronchial carcinoma.

Imaging Signs

▶ **Modality of choice**
Primarily radiography, although false negatives are common, especially in the spine and pelvis (complex or superimposing anatomy) • If malignancy is suspected despite negative radiographic findings, obtain MRI or CT studies • To search for metastases in patients with a known primary tumor, scintigraphy or whole-body MRI is recommended, depending on primary malignancy.

▶ **Radiographic findings**
Location: axial skeleton (regions with hematopoietic bone marrow) • Rarely peripheral: most common cause is bronchial carcinoma.
Three forms:
– Osteolytic with permeative and/or "moth-eaten" destruction, cortical destruction (Lodwick II and III).
– Osteoblastic with sclerosis of the bone.
– Mixed osteolytic/osteoblastic.
Vertebral column: destruction of the pedicle of the vertebral arch (AP view, pathologic vertebral body fracture) • Typical osteoclastic metastases: bronchial carcinoma, renal carcinoma • Typical osteoblastic metastases: prostate carcinoma, breast carcinoma (may be primarily purely osteolytic).

▶ **MRI findings**
Osteolytic metastases: Hypointense foci on T1-weighted SE images • Hyperintense on fat-saturated sequences (e.g., STIR) • Isointense or hyperintense on T2-weighted TSE images • Markedly enhancing after contrast administration.
Osteoblastic metastases: Hypointense on T1-weighted SE images • Isointense or slightly hyperintense on fat-saturated images • Hypointense on T2-weighted TSE images • Usually moderately enhancing after contrast administration.

▶ **Nuclear medicine**
Accumulation of ^{99m}Tc, especially in osteoblastic and mixed lytic/blastic lesions • Osteolytic metastases, especially renal carcinoma and bronchial carcinoma, may produce normal findings on scintigraphy.

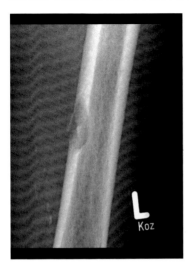

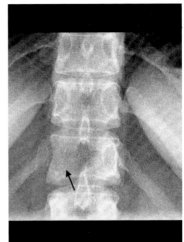

Fig. 1.23 An 89-year-old woman. Radiograph showing cortical metastasis in left femur. Cortical destruction. Primary tumor unknown.

Fig. 1.24 A 34-year-old woman with metastasizing breast carcinoma. AP spinal radiograph showing destruction of the right pedicle of the vertebral arch at T12.

Clinical Aspects

▶ **Typical presentation**
  Pain • Weight loss in patients with generalized metastatic disease.
▶ **Treatment options**
  For solitary lesions, wide resection and endoprosthesis • For generalized disease, chemotherapy and/or radiation therapy according to primary tumor • Vertebroplasty to treat vertebral involvement.
▶ **Course and prognosis**
  Usually unfavorable since bone metastasis indicates hematogenous seeding.
▶ **What does the clinician want to know?**
  Location • Size • Lytic/blastic activity • Stability of the bone: unstable if more than 50% of the transverse diameter is affected or if more than 50% of the cortex is eroded • Multiple foci • Cortical breakthrough • Pathologic fracture • Findings requiring further investigation, preferably by MRI: soft-tissue component, encircling of nerves and vessels, joint involvement.

Differential Diagnosis

Benign bone tumor	– Geographic, solitary lesion
	– No cortical breakthrough
	– Sclerotic rim (e.g., bone cyst, aneurysmal bone cyst)

Osteoma	– No accumulation on scintigraphy, unlike osteoblastic metastases
Primary bone tumor	– Often cannot be distinguished – Solitary focus and tumor matrix calcifications tend to suggest a primary bone tumor
Multiple myeloma	– Multiple, usually similarly shaped, punched-out defects (salt-and-pepper skull) – Paraproteins on electrophoresis
Lymphoma	– Primary lymphoma (rare) – Secondary lymphoma in generalized disease – Difficult to distinguish
Recent osteoporotic vertebral compression fracture	– Often difficult to distinguish radiographically from neoplastic vertebral compression fracture in the absence of trauma when there is a solitary spontaneous fracture – Both entities demonstrate tracer accumulation on bone scans – Additional studies: MRI: band-like marrow edema, increased diffusion; CT: no osteolysis, no soft-tissue density

Tips and Pitfalls

False-negative result on radiography (at least 40% of the bone structure must be destroyed before an osteolytic lesion is detectable); if there is clinical suspicion, refer for CT or MRI ● Tracer accumulation on bone scans may be caused by degenerative disease or osteoporotic collapse; radiographic follow-up, CT, or MRI studies are always necessary.

Selected References

Baur A. Diffusion-weighted imaging of bone marrow: current status. Eur Radiol 2003; 13(7): 1699–1708

Ghanem N, Uhl M, Brink I, et al. Diagnostic value of MRI in comparison to scintigraphy, PET, MS-CT and PET/CT for the detection of metastases of bone. Eur J Radiol 2005; 55(1): 41–55

Krishnamurthy GT, Tubis M, Hiss J, Blahd WH. Distribution pattern of metastatic bone disease. JAMA 1977; 237(23): 2504–2506

Ollivier L, Gerber S, Vanel D, Brisse H, Leclère J. Improving the interpretation of bone marrow imaging in cancer patients. Cancer Imaging 2006; 6: 194–198

Stacy GS, Mahal RS, Peabody TD. Staging of bone tumors: a review with illustrative examples. AJR Am J Roentgenol 2006; 186(4): 967–976

Steinborn MM, Heuck AF, Tiling R, Bruegel M, Gauger L, Reiser MF. Whole-body bone marrow MRI in patients with metastatic disease to the skeletal system. J Comput Assist Tomogr 1999; 23(1): 123–129

Thrall JH, Ellis BI. Skeletal metastases. Radiol Clin North Am 1996; 25: 1155–1170

Toomayan GA, Robertson F, Major NM. Lower extremity compartmental anatomy: clinical relevance to radiologists. Skeletal Radiol 2005; 34(6): 307–313

Vanel D, Bittoun J, Tardivon A. MRI of bone metastases. Eur Radiol 1998; 8(8): 1345–1351

Definition

▶ **Epidemiology**
Most common primary malignant bone tumor ● Incidence is 2–3 in 1 million ●
Peak incidence: 10–25 and 60–80 years.

▶ **Etiology, pathophysiology, pathogenesis**
Histologically characteristic osteoid/bone production by sarcomatous osteoblasts ● Primary or secondary degeneration, e.g., Paget osteosarcoma or after radiation therapy ● "Classic intramedullary osteosarcoma" is most prevalent type
(90%).
Variants:
 – Intraosseous telangiectatic osteosarcoma: cystic, blood-filled spaces ● Islands
 of osteoid-forming tumor cells ● Usually affects adolescents and young adults.
 – Primary multicentric osteosarcoma: debatable whether primarily multicentric or early bone metastasis ● Usually purely osteoblastic foci.
 – Other rare forms: intraosseous small-cell osteosarcoma, osteoblastoma-like
 osteosarcoma, low-grade osteosarcoma.
Surface osteosarcomas:
 – Parosteal osteosarcoma: usually low-grade tumor ● Rarely with a high-grade
 dedifferentiated component or osteochondroma-like, low-grade parosteal os-
 teosarcoma ● Arises from outer cortical surface ● Second through fourth decades.
 – Periosteal osteosarcoma: high-grade tumor ● Predominantly chondroblastic ●
 Arises in the periosteum ● Mainly occurs in the 2nd decade of life.
 – High-grade surface osteosarcoma: superficial lesion ● Lies on cortex ● Histo-
 logically indistinguishable from classic osteosarcoma.
 – Extraosseous osteosarcoma: often after radiation therapy ● Very rare ● Older
 patient age.

Imaging Signs

▶ **Modality of choice**
Radiography ● MRI.
▶ **Pathognomonic findings**
Bone tumor with mixed cell population (predominantly osteoblastic, some osteolytic), metadiaphyseal location, knee involvement, malignant periosteal reaction, manifestation in 2nd decade.
▶ **Radiographic/CT findings**
Classic osteosarcoma: Tumor matrix is typically ossified ● Usually mixed osteo-
blastic/osteolytic ● Poorly defined bone lesion ● Potentially aggressive, purely
lytic or blastic lesion (Lodwick II–III) ● Usually malignant periosteal changes
(spiculation, Codman triangle) ● Dense soft-tissue component and cortical destruction often found ● Location: usually metaphyseal or metadiaphyseal on
long tubular bones (60% near the knee joint, 10% involve proximal humerus) ●
Extraosseous, partially ossified tumor mass often visible on radiographs.

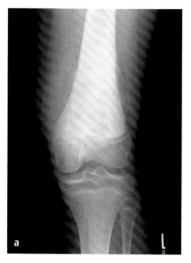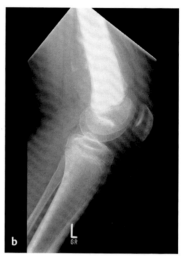

Fig. 1.25 a, b   Osteosarcoma. Radiograph of the left femur in two planes. A 16-year-old boy with osteosarcoma of the distal tibia. Typical aggressive growth pattern with extensive periosteal reactions (spiculation producing "sunburst" appearance). Ossifications in the surrounding soft tissues.

Telangiectatic osteosarcoma: Resembles aneurysmal bone cyst • Expansile, lytic nature • Usually geographic • Cortical destruction and pathologic fracture (50% femur, 25% tibia) are common findings • Metadiaphyseal location • Periosteal reaction commonly seen.

Periosteal osteosarcoma: Lies on outer cortical surface • Calcified central portions near the cortex • Linear mineralization • Occasional cortical erosion or reactive thickening • Predilection for diaphyseal location on femur and tibia • Differential diagnosis: juxtacortical chondroma/chondrosarcoma.

Parosteal osteosarcoma: At the posterior surface of the distal femur • Usually marked central sclerosis (mineralized matrix) • Cortical thickening • Poorly defined • Differential diagnosis: cortical irregularity (periosteal desmoid) of gastrocnemius attachment site.

High-grade surface osteosarcoma: Diaphyseal location • Resembles periosteal osteosarcoma, although generally less mineralized.

Extraosseous osteosarcoma: Soft-tissue calcification tends to be central, unlike in myositis ossificans • Predilection for buttocks and thighs.

▶ **MRI findings**

Helpful for differential diagnosis (solid space-occupying mass, cystic) and evaluating extent (resectability: neurovascular invasion, joint collapse).

Classic osteosarcoma: Hypointense intramedullary signal on T1-weighted SE images • Hyperintense on fat-saturated images • Hypointense or hyperintense on T2-weighted SE images depending on degree of mineralization (osteoblastic

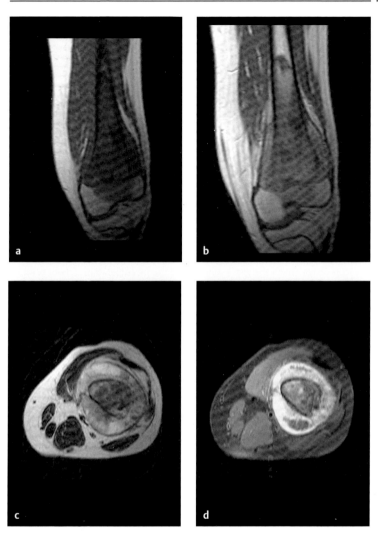

Fig. 1.26 a–d MRI of same patient.
a Coronal noncontrast T1-weighted SE image.
b Coronal T1-weighted SE image after contrast administration. Inhomogeneous enhancement of medullary space and soft-tissue component.
c Axial noncontrast T2-weighted TSE sequence. Extensive tumor infiltration of the soft tissues around the femoral shaft. Femoral vessels are not encircled.
d Axial fat-saturated T1-weighted SE sequence after contrast administration.

components: hypointense) ● Inhomogeneous but strongly enhancing ● Paraosseous soft-tissue component often seen.

Telangiectatic osteosarcoma: Fluid–fluid levels due to hemorrhage ● Solid, enhancing tumor components distinguish it from aneurysmal bone cyst.

Surface osteosarcomas: Soft-tissue tumors lying on the cortex ● Evidence of medullary space invasion, which carries a poor prognosis ● Periosteal osteosarcoma: extremely high signal intensity, lobulated appearance, septal contrast enhancement resembling a chondroid tumor.

▶ **Nuclear medicine**
Bone scans show high levels of tracer accumulation ● Detection of skip lesions and bone metastases in the rest of the skeletal system (alternatively, whole-body MRI).

Clinical Aspects

▶ **Typical presentation**
Pain ● In children, pain is often referred to an adjacent joint—always obtain radiographs of adjacent bones.

▶ **Treatment options**
Preoperative chemotherapy ● Wide resection or amputation ● Postoperative chemotherapy (to prevent distant metastasis).

▶ **Course and prognosis**
Depending on tumor type and response to preoperative chemotherapy: 5-year survival rate of 50–80% ● In 10–20% distant metastasis at the time of diagnosis ● More favorable prognosis for parosteal and low-grade osteosarcomas ● Metastasis usually involves lungs and bones.

▶ **What does the clinician want to know?**
Extent of tumor ● Relationship to neurovascular bundle ● Joint collapse ● Epiphyseal involvement (detectable on MRI in 80%, on radiographs in 15%!) ● Skip lesions – always obtain images of entire extremity, coronal noncontrast T1-weighted SE sequence ● Response to preoperative chemotherapy (MRI: decreased tumor size, areas of necrosis without contrast administration) – if no response, adjust chemotherapy regimen.

Differential Diagnosis

Ewing sarcoma	– Usually not mineralized
	– Occurs at an earlier age
Chondrosarcoma	– Typical chondroid calcifications may be found
	– Age 40–60 years
Metastases	– Often cannot be distinguished
	– Rarely occur in children
	– Usually no ossification of tumor matrix

Osteoma	– Sharply defined – No periosteal reaction – No cortical breakthrough – Usually small, round lesion – Typical location: paranasal sinuses
Osteomyelitis	– May be difficult to distinguish – Minimal/no soft-tissue component – No tumor matrix – No bony spicules
Cortical desmoid	– Eccentrically located on the cortex of the distal femoral metaphysis – Sharply defined – Negative bone scan
Fibrosarcoma/MFH	– Differential diagnosis especially to distinguish from telangiectatic osteosarcoma on radiographs, since lesions are also lytic; on MRI no blood-filled spaces, but solid tissue
Aneurysmal bone cyst	– Differential diagnosis for telangiectatic osteosarcoma – More aggressive growth pattern – Enhancement only of periphery or septa on MRI – No enhancing nodular or solid structures

Tips and Pitfalls

– Delayed diagnosis can result from failure to evaluate adjacent joints/regions or misdiagnosis of a pathologic fracture (e.g., while playing) as traumatic.
– Insufficient resection/therapy can result from missing skip lesions during preoperative assessment or inadequate staging (thoracic CT, bone scan) – solitary lung metastases may be resected with a chance of healing.
– Biopsy path should be positioned within the surgical route so that the needle track can be removed during definitive surgery.

Selected References

Andresen KJ, Sundaram M, Unii KK, Sim FH. Imaging features of low grade central osteosarcoma of the long bones and pelvis. Skeletal Radiol 2004; 33(7): 373–379

Brisse H, Ollivier L, Edeline V, et al. Imaging of malignant tumors of the long bones in children. Monitoring response to neoadjuvant chemotherapy and preoperative assessment. Pediatr Radiol 2004; 34(8): 595–605

Gladish GW, Sabloff BM, Munden RF, Truong MT, Erasmus JJ, Chasen MH. Primary thoracic sarcomas. Radiographics 2002; 22(3): 621–637

Saifuddin A. The accuracy of imaging in the local staging of appendicular osteosarcoma. Skeletal Radiol 2002; 31(4): 191–201

Suresh S, Saifuddin A. Radiological appearances of appendicular osteosarcoma: a comprehensive pictorial review. Clin Radiol 2007; 62(4): 314–323

Definition

▶ **Epidemiology**
Second most common malignant bone tumor • Peak incidence: 30–50 years •
Men affected twice as often as women.

▶ **Etiology, pathophysiology, pathogenesis**
Malignant bone tumor whose cells form cartilage but not osteoid • Occurs as
primary or secondary disease after radiation therapy or from malignant degeneration of primary benign bone tumor (enchondromatosis, Ollier disease, hereditary exostosis).

Imaging Signs

▶ **Modality of choice**
Conventional radiographs (at least two planes).

▶ **Pathognomonic findings**
Aggressively growing osteolytic tumor • Areas of chondroid calcification • Enhancing rings and arcs on MRI.

▶ **Radiographic/CT findings**
Usually centrally located near the metaphysis of long bones as well as in the pel-
vis and ribs • Rarely subperiosteal, eccentric, or extraosseous.
Findings by tumor grade:
  – Low-grade: smoothly bordered lucency with central, popcorn-like chondroid
    calcifications • Scalloping of the cortex (similar to enchondroma).
  – Intermediate and high-grade: moth-eaten or permeative growth pattern with
    or without chondroid calcifications • Cortical breakthrough • Soft-tissue
    component with calcifications • Periosteal reactions possible.

▶ **MRI findings**
Hypointense on T1-weighted SE images • Hyperintense on T2-weighted SE and
fat-saturated images • Arcs of contrast enhancement, consistent with the lobulated structure of the cartilage matrix, are typical of chondroid tumors.

Clinical Aspects

▶ **Typical presentation**
Sudden onset of dull pain.

▶ **Treatment options**
Resection • Responds poorly to radiation therapy • Effectiveness of adjuvant
chemotherapy remains uncertain • Large, axial chondroid tumors that are active
or aggressive on radiography must be completely removed with or without evidence of malignancy • Peripheral chondroid tumors (e.g., phalanges) tend to be
benign.

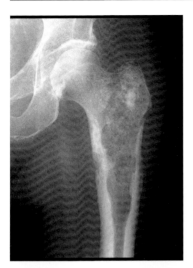

Fig. 1.27 A 64-year-old patient with progressive pain in the left thigh. Radiograph showing lesion with aggressive, "motheaten," osteolytic destruction in the metaphyseal/diaphyseal region of the left proximal femur. Grade III chondrosarcoma.

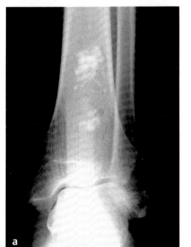

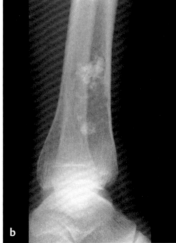

Fig. 1.28 a, b Chondrosarcoma in a 61-year-old patient. **a** AP and **b** lateral radiographs. "Bubbly" osteolytic lesion in the distal tibia shaft. Popcorn-like calcifications. The lesion has rather irregular borders with normal bone, possibly indicating malignancy. Grade I chondrosarcoma. Differential diagnosis includes benign enchondroma and bone infarct.

▶ **Course and prognosis**

Slow-growing lesion ● Hematological seeding in the lungs is rare and occurs only in tumors near the center of the body ● 10-year survival rate depends on histological grade: grade I: 40–80%; grade II: 40–60%; grade III: 15–35%.

▶ **What does the clinician want to know?**

Joint collapse ● Relationship to neighboring structures (vessels, nerves) ● Skip metastases

Differential Diagnosis

Enchondroma	– Differentiation from grade I chondrosarcoma is not always possible radiographically or even histologically
Metastases	– Differentiation often impossible, especially in the absence of chondroid calcifications
Lymphoma	– No chondroid calcifications
Osteosarcoma	– More sclerotic components

Tips and Pitfalls

Confusing low-grade chondrosarcoma and enchondroma, resulting in overtreatment or undertreatment ● Always obtain histology if pain is present.

Selected References

Cummings JE, Ellzey JA, Heck RK. Imaging of bone sarcomas [review]. J Natl Compr Canc Netw 2007; 5(4): 438–447

Murphey MD, Walker EA, Wilson AJ, Kransdorf MJ, Temple HT, Gannon FH. From the archives of the AFIP: Imaging of primary chondrosarcoma: radiologic-pathologic correlation. Radiographics 2003; 23(5): 1245–1278

Patil S, de Silva MV, Crossan J, Reid R. Chondrosarcoma of small bones of the hand. J Hand Surg Br 2003; 28(6): 602–608

Definition

▶ **Epidemiology**
Second most common malignant bone tumor in children ● Age 9–18 ● Ratio of boys to girls is 3:2.

▶ **Etiology, pathophysiology, pathogenesis**
Highly malignant tumor arising from the bone marrow ● No production of tumor matrix.

Imaging Signs

▶ **Modality of choice**
MRI ● Radiographs in two planes.

▶ **Pathognomonic findings**
Aggressively growing bone tumor found in children and adolescents ● Predominantly osteolytic ● Metadiaphyseal location ● Malignant periosteal reaction ● Soft-tissue component.

▶ **Radiographic findings**
Predominantly located near the metaphysis/diaphysis of long bones (60%) ● Less often in flat bones (pelvis) or vertebral bodies ● Moth-eaten or permeative destruction (Lodwick II–III) ● Usually osteolytic ● Sometimes also osteoblastic intraosseous components ● Often cortical breakthrough with soft-tissue component which is usually very large in flat bones ● Periosteal reactions are a common finding: spiculation (periosteal new bone formation radiating into the soft tissues) and onion-skin periosteal ossification ● Codman triangle: elevated, ossified periosteum at the margin of the subperiosteal tumor ● "Sunburst" appearance: periosteal new bone along the Sharpey fibers between the periosteum and cortex.

▶ **MRI findings**
Especially suitable for demonstrating the full extent of the tumor ● Good visualization of the extent of the tumor in the medullary cavity on T1-weighted SE (hypointense) and fat-saturated (hyperintense) images ● Strongly enhancing ● Loss of signal intensity possible in central areas of necrosis ● Demonstration of skip lesions – always image long bones in their entirety.

▶ **CT findings**
Sensitive demonstration of extent of bone destruction or a pathologic fracture ● Staging, especially for detection of lung metastases.

▶ **Nuclear medicine**
Isotope uptake more marked in tumors with large sclerotic components than in purely osteolytic tumors ● Staging: detection of bone metastases.

Clinical Aspects

▶ **Typical presentation**
Pain and swelling at the site of the tumor ● Pain often referred to adjacent joint ● Common symptoms: fever, anemia, leukocytosis, increased ESR ● Erythema and increased local warmth ● Complaints arising from compression of adjacent

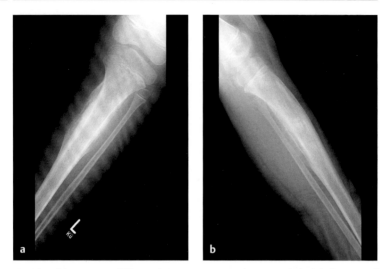

Fig. 1.29 a, b A 10-year-old boy with Ewing sarcoma in the proximal tibial shaft. **a** AP and **b** lateral radiographs. Highly aggressive, permeative growth pattern corresponding to a Lodwick grade III lesion with marked lamellar periosteal reaction, interrupted in places.

structures • Hematogenous pulmonary metastases, bone metastases, lymph node metastases.

▶ **Treatment options**

First, neoadjuvant polychemotherapy with or without local radiation therapy • Radical tumor resection with the aim of limb salvage • Subsequent adjuvant chemotherapy.

▶ **Course and prognosis**

Prognosis depends on primary tumor resectability, metastasis, and tumor chemosensitivity.

▶ **What does the clinician want to know?**

Tumor volume • Tumor operability: neurovascular invasion, extracompartmental spread • Distant metastases.

Differential Diagnosis

Osteomyelitis	– Clinical and radiographic findings are similar
	– No paraosseous soft-tissue component on MRI studies
	– Detection of abscess on MRI
	– Possible sequestra on CT
	– More regular lamellated periosteal reaction
Osteosarcoma	– May be impossible to distinguish
	– Same age group
	– Parosteal calcifications in the soft-tissue component

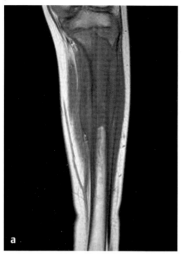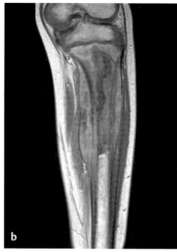

Fig. 1.30 a, b Ewing sarcoma in the same patient. MRI **a** before and **b** after contrast administration. Entire medullary cavity has been infiltrated, with cortical breakthrough in a paraosseous direction. Marked infiltration of the soft tissues.

Eosinophilic granuloma	– Usually difficult to distinguish
	– Same age group
	– Lesions tend to be geographic (Lodwick I, more aggressive forms possible)
	– Usually no soft-tissue component
Other neoplasias	– Lymphoma with primary osseous manifestation
	– Embryonal rhabdomyosarcoma
	– Reticulosarcoma
	– Multiple myeloma
	– Metastasis

Tips and Pitfalls

Failure to image the tumor-bearing portion of the bone in patients with pain referred to an adjacent joint, resulting in delayed diagnosis • Missing skip lesions.

Selected References

Aoki J, Inoue T, Tomiyoshi K, et al. Nuclear imaging of bone tumors: FDG-PET [review]. Semin Musculoskelet Radiol 2001; 5(2): 183–187

Brisse H, Ollivier L, Edeline V, et al. Imaging of malignant tumours of the long bones in children: monitoring response to neoadjuvant chemotherapy and preoperative assessment [review]. Pediatr Radiol 2004; 34(8): 595–605

Carvajal R, Meyers P. Ewing's sarcoma and primitive neuroectodermal family of tumors [review]. Hematol Oncol Clin North Am 2005; 19(3): 501–525, vi–vii

Tumors

Definition

▶ **Epidemiology**
Incidence is 3 in 100 000 ● Usually manifests after age 40 ● Peak incidence at around age 60.

▶ **Etiology, pathophysiology, pathogenesis**
Aggressive non-Hodgkin lymphoma ● Infiltration of bone marrow by atypical monoclonal plasma cells ● Nest-like and/or diffuse pattern of involvement ● Replacement of hematopoietic bone marrow ● Destruction of bone tissue with potential for spontaneous fracture ● Formation of monoclonal immunoglobulins or light chains by degenerated plasma cells ("paraprotein" detectable on electrophoresis).

Imaging Signs

▶ **Modality of choice**
Radiography ● Radiography increasingly supplanted by whole-body MRI (superior sensitivity) ● Alternatively, whole-body multislice CT.

▶ **Radiographic findings**
Radiographic skeletal survey: skull bones, humeri, spine, pelvis, femora, and hemithorax ● In highly diffuse pattern of involvement: osteoporotic striations ● In focal pattern of involvement: well-defined osteolytic lesions ● Predilection for axial skeleton, especially spine and pelvis ● Typical appearance on skull images: "salt-and-pepper skull" (multiple, relatively similarly shaped osteolytic lesions) ● 50–70% false-negative findings on conventional radiographs ● Complications: pathologic fracture, especially involving the spine.
Solitary plasmacytoma: Isolated focus of plasma cells ● Relatively well-defined solitary osteolytic lesion ● Paraosseous tumor component usually clearly visible ● Generally transforms within 2–10 years into multiple myeloma.
POEMS: Sclerosing form of plasmacytoma with polyneuropathy and skin changes.

▶ **MRI findings**
Most sensitive study for depicting bone marrow involvement ● Diffuse pattern: diffusely reduced signal intensity on T1-weighted SE sequences with increased signal intensity after contrast administration, usually increased signal intensity on fat-suppressed sequences (e.g., STIR) ● Focal pattern: circumscribed areas that appear hypointense on T1-weighted SE sequences (exhibiting increased signal intensity after contrast administration) and hyperintense on fat-suppressed sequences ● Low level of infiltration and diffuse pattern of involvement (< 20 vol% plasma cells in bone marrow): signal intensity corresponds to that of normal bone marrow (hyperintense on T1-weighted SE and hypointense on fat-saturated sequences) ● Complications: pathologic fracture, paraosseous tumor components, spinal-cord compression ● Whole-body MRI whenever possible to assess entire medullary cavity.

▶ **CT findings**
Show extent of bone destruction ● Estimate fracture risk ● Whole-body multislice CT with low-dose protocol (120 kV, 100 mAs) is increasingly replacing radiographic skeletal survey, given its clearly superior sensitivity for detection of osteolytic lesions.

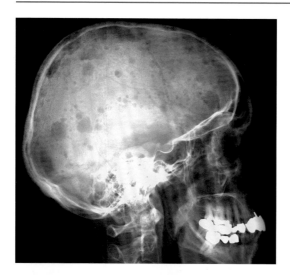

Fig. 1.31 A 46-year-old woman with multiple myeloma and multiple sharply defined osteolytic lesions in the calvarial bones.

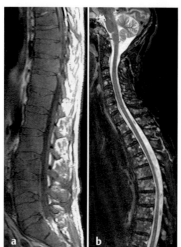

Fig. 1.32 a, b **a** A 53-year-old man with myeloma and diffuse involvement of the spine. MRI, T1-weighted SE sequence. Markedly reduced signal intensity indicating hypercellularity of the bone marrow and decreased fat content. **b** Multifocal infiltration of a patient with multiple myeloma showing multifocal hyperintensities on a STIR sequence.

Clinical Aspects

▶ **Typical presentation**

Bone pain • Generalized symptoms including fatigue and weight loss • Monoclonal immunoglobulins in blood plasma and/or urine: "M gradient" on serum protein electrophoresis, light chains (Bence Jones proteins) in urine • Dramatically increased ESR ● Anemia ● Hypercalcemia ● β_2-Microglobulin as a marker for presence of tumor ● Complications: spontaneous fractures, renal insufficiency due to toxic effect of light chains on renal tubules, hypercalcemic crises, infections, cytopenia. Staging according to Durie and Salmon system using laboratory values (hemoglobin, calcium, paraprotein, creatinine) and radiological findings (radiography/MRI).

► **Treatment options**
Stage I: "watch and wait" ● Stage II–III: high-dose chemotherapy followed by autologous or, in rare situations, allogenic stem-cell transplantation ● Prophylactic bisphosphonates (inhibit osteoclast activity).

► **Course and prognosis**
Slow-growing "smoldering myeloma" in 10% (survival rate of about 10 years) ● Average survival of 3–5 years in manifest multiple myeloma.

► **What does the clinician want to know?**
Extent of skeletal involvement (number of foci, diffuse infiltration) ● Estimation of fracture risk ● Complications.

Differential Diagnosis

Osteolytic bone metastases	– Bronchial carcinoma, renal cell carcinoma, etc.
	– Often impossible to distinguish
	– Laboratory tests!
Osteoporosis	– Often impossible to distinguish radiographically
	– Diagnostic evidence: normal marrow signal on MRI

Tips and Pitfalls

Misdiagnosing multiple myeloma as osteoporosis ● Obtain MRI studies if conventional radiographic findings are negative ● Mistaking a pathologic fracture for an osteoporotic fracture.

Selected References

Baur A. Magnetic resonance imaging as a supplement for the clinical staging system of Durie and Salmon? Cancer 2002; 95(6): 1334–1345

Baur-Melnyk A, Buhmann S, Dürr HR, Reiser M. Role of MRI for the diagnosis and prognosis of multiple myeloma. Eur J Radiol 2005; 55(1): 56–63

Durie BG, Kyle RA, Belch A, Bensinger W, Blade J. Myeloma management guidelines: a consensus report from the Scientific Advisors of the International Myeloma Foundation. Hematol J 2003; 4(6): 379–398, erratum in Hematol J 2004; 5(3): 285

Stäbler A, Baur A, Bartl R, Munker R, Lamerz R, Reiser M. Contrast enhancement and quantitative signal analysis in MR imaging of multiple myeloma: assessment of focal and diffuse growth patterns in marrow correlated with biopsies and survival rates. AJR Am J Roentgenol 1996; 167(4): 1029–1036

Van de Berg BC, Lecouvert F, Michaux L, et al. Stage I multiple myeloma: value of MRI of the bone marrow in the determination of the prognosis. Radiology 1996; 201(1): 243–246

Definition

▶ **Epidemiology**
  Any age ● Peak incidence: 5th through 7th decades of life.
▶ **Etiology, pathophysiology, pathogenesis**
  Primary lymphoma of bone is rare (3%) ● Usually secondary tumor in a context of generalized lymphoma: non-Hodgkin lymphoma (40%), Hodgkin disease (20%).

Imaging Signs

▶ **Modality of choice**
  Radiography ● MRI.
▶ **Radiographic findings**
  Primary lymphoma of bone usually involves metaphysis or diaphysis of long tubular bones ● Secondary lymphoma of bone usually affects the axial skeleton, especially the spine and pelvis ● Moth-eaten or permeative destruction ● Pattern of growth varies: osteolytic, mixed lytic/blastic, or predominantly sclerotic (Lodwick II–III) ● Possible soft-tissue component ● Typical finding of ivory vertebrae (highly osteoblastic vertebral bodies).
▶ **MRI findings**
  Most sensitive study ● Shows extent of bone marrow infiltration.
  Focal lesions: Mainly in high-grade malignant lymphoma ● Hypointense on T1-weighted SE images ● From isointense to hyperintense on T2-weighted TSE images ● Sclerotic lesions are hypointense on T2-weighted SE images, hyperintense on fat-suppressed sequences (e.g., STIR), enhancing after contrast administration.
  Diffuse bone marrow infiltration: Mainly in low-grade malignant lymphoma ● Signal intensity usually unaltered given the low interstitial distribution of lymphoma cells in bone marrow ● Extensive diffuse pattern of involvement shows homogeneously low signal intensity on T1-weighted SE images, hyperintense on fat-saturated sequences, with tumor enhancement after contrast administration.
▶ **CT findings**
  Extent of bone destruction: osteolytic, mixed lytic/blastic, or purely osteosclerotic.
▶ **Nuclear medicine/PET-CT**
  Foci of tracer accumulation.

Fig. 1.33 A 64-year-old woman with primary non-Hodgkin lymphoma of bone. Axial CT scan reveals extensive destruction with mixed lytic and permeative appearance as well as sclerotic components in the left ilium.

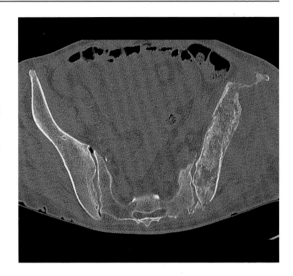

Clinical Aspects

▶ **Typical presentation**
Local pain ● Pathologic fracture possible ● Generalized symptoms in secondary lymphoma of bone: lymph node enlargement, hepatosplenomegaly.

▶ **Treatment options**
Radiation therapy ● Adjuvant chemotherapy ● Surgical stabilization if risk of fracture.

▶ **Course and prognosis**
Depend on subtype and stage at diagnosis ● In Hodgkin disease 70 % recover with combined radiation therapy and chemotherapy.

▶ **What does the clinician want to know?**
Solitary lesion (primary lymphoma of bone) ● Secondary involvement in systemic lymphoma ● Size ● Osteoclastic/osteoblastic ● Stability.

Differential Diagnosis

If underlying disease is known, differential diagnosis is not problematic.

Metastases of small-cell tumors	– Impossible to distinguish radiologically – Multiple foci
Primary bone tumor	– Virtually impossible to distinguish
Chronic osteomyelitis	– Usually wide sclerotic rim around lytic lesion – Cortical thickening – Patient history and laboratory tests

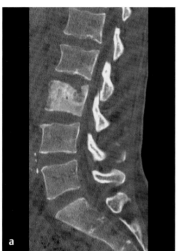

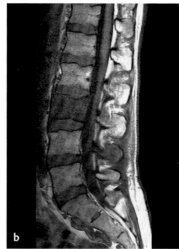

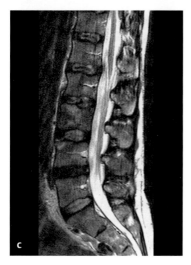

Fig. 1.34 a–c   A 38-year-old woman with anaplastic non-Hodgkin lymphoma and secondary involvement of L3.
a   16-slice CT, sagittal reconstruction. Predominantly sclerotic density with vertebral compression fracture involving superior end plate.
b   T1-weighted SE sequence. Infiltrated vertebral body is markedly hypointense compared with healthy bone marrow.
c   T2-weighted TSE sequence. Hypointense signal in L3 resulting from new bone formation.

Tips and Pitfalls

Missing small lesions on radiographs • Mistaking the lesion for metastasis.

Selected References

Davies AN, Salisbury JR, Dobbs HJ. Primary bone lymphoma: report of an unusual case with a review of the literature [review]. Clin Oncol (R Coll Radiol) 1994; 6(6):411–412

Dürr HR, Müller PE, Hiller E, Baur A, Jansson V, Refior HJ. Malignant lymphoma of bone. Arch Orthop Trauma Surg 2002; 122(1): 10–16

Gill P, Wenger DE, Inwards DJ. Primary lymphomas of bone [review]. Clin Lymphoma Myeloma 2005; 6(2): 140–142

Krishnan A, Shirkhoda A, Tehranzadeh J, Armin AR, Irwin R, Les K. Primary bone lymphoma: radiographic–MR imaging correlation [review]. Radiographics 2003; 23(6): 1371–1383; discussion 1384–1387

Malloy PC, Fishman EK, Magid D. Lymphoma of bone, muscle, and skin: CT findings [review]. AJR Am J Roentgenol 1992; 159(4): 805–809

Miguez Sanchez C, Hebrero ML, Mesa C, Villanego I, Sanchez Calzado JA, Errazquin L. Primary bone lymphoma [review]. Clin Transl Oncol 2006; 8(3): 221–224

Schmidt GP, Schoenberg SO, Reiser MF, Baur-Melnyk A. Whole-body MR imaging of bone marrow [review]. Eur J Radiol 2005; 55(1): 33–40

Definition

▶ **Epidemiology**
The spine is the most common site of bone metastases (64%).
▶ **Etiology, pathophysiology, pathogenesis**
Usually hematogenous metastasis of various primary tumors, e.g., breast carcinoma, prostate carcinoma, renal cell carcinoma, multiple myeloma, lymphoma •
Vertebral metastases occur via the vertebral venous plexus, the lymphatic system, or by direct invasion into surrounding tissues.

Imaging Signs

▶ **Modality of choice**
Radiography • MRI.
▶ **Pathognomonic findings**
Radiography: asymmetrical vertebral body collapse, pedicular destruction • CT: osseous destruction with soft-tissue density • MRI: complete signal alteration in bone marrow of entire vertebra, soft-tissue component.
▶ **Radiographic findings**
Decrease in vertebral body height • Typical finding of asymmetrical collapse • Pedicular destruction on AP images • Osseous destruction • Differentiation from spontaneous osteoporotic fractures often difficult in the absence of unequivocal signs.
▶ **CT findings**
Better demonstration of osseous destruction and malignant new bone formation • Soft-tissue density in osteolytic lesions • Paraosseous soft-tissue components may be present.
Risk of vertebral fracture with lytic destruction of:
 – more than 50% of a thoracic vertebra (T1–T10).
 – more than 25% of a thoracic vertebra with costovertebral destruction.
 – more than 35% of a thoracolumbar vertebra (T11–L5).
 – more than 20% of a thoracolumbar vertebra (T11–L5) if additional involvement of posterior elements.
▶ **MRI findings**
Vertebral collapse with signal alterations typical of tumor • Hypointense on T1-weighted SE images • Hyperintense, heterogeneous in places, on T2-weighted SE and fat-saturated images • Enhancement after contrast administration • Posterior vertebral wall often convex • Diffusion-weighted images (hyperintense) may be helpful.
▶ **Nuclear medicine**
Metastases usually show strong, early accumulation of ^{99m}Tc • Highly sensitive, but not very specific (accumulation also occurs with recent osteoporotic collapse) • Other foci are often found, supporting a diagnosis of metastasis.

Fig. 1.35 Neoplastic vertebral body fracture in a 44-year-old man with multiple myeloma. CT scan showing pathologic vertebral fractures of L2 and L5. Marked osteolytic destruction of L5.

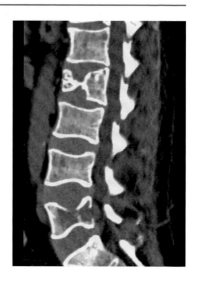

Clinical Aspects

▶ **Typical presentation**

Local pain • Narrowing or infiltration of vertebral canal may cause neurologic symptoms.

▶ **Treatment options**

Surgical management of acute instability and neurologic symptoms • Possible surgical stabilization and decompression for (impending) fractures • Sample collection for histology • Radiation therapy • Bisphosphonates • Percutaneous CT-guided vertebroplasty.

▶ **Course and prognosis**

Mortality depends on overall situation (additional metastases, comorbidity, type of underlying tumor) • Prognosis with bone metastasis is very poor.

▶ **What does the clinician want to know?**

Type and extent of loss of vertebral body height • Extent of tumor infiltration and osseous destruction • Involvement of posterior margin of vertebral body • Involvement of posterior elements • Vertebral canal compromise by tumor infiltration or bone • Spinal-cord compression • Differentiate from osteoporotic fracture.

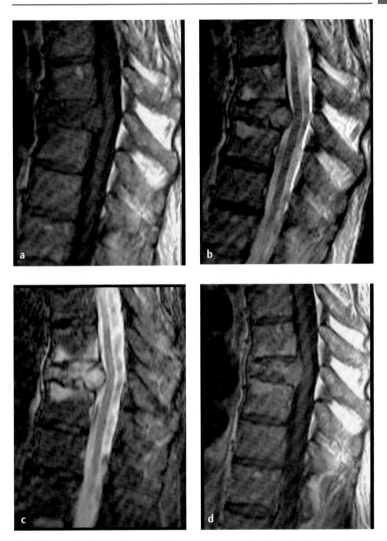

Fig. 1.36 a–d A 64-year-old man with increasing pain in the thoracic spine. Spinal MRI showing fracture of T8. Convex posterior vertebral wall typical of malignancy. The search for a tumor resulted in identification of a metastasis of a previously undetected bronchial carcinoma. **a** T1-weighted SE sequence. Hypointense signal throughout the thoracic spine. **b** T2-weighted TSE. Hyperintense signal. **c** Fat-saturated STIR image. **d** Enhancement after contrast administration.

Tumors

Differential Diagnosis

Osteoporotic fracture	– Radiography: symmetrical collapse, no osseous destruction
	– CT: no soft-tissue densities in fractured vertebral body; intraosseous vacuum phenomenon may be seen
	– MRI: older fractures demonstrate normal marrow signal; acute osteoporotic fractures usually show band-like edema along the fractured vertebral end plate or more extensive edema, although small islands of normal fatty marrow are generally still present. No epidural soft-tissue masses.
Spondylodiskitis	– Intensely enhancing vertebral disk
	– Disk space: markedly hyperintense on T2-weighted SE images
	– Destruction of vertebral end plates on T1-weighted SE images
	– Inflammatory edema on both sides of vertebral disk

Tips and Pitfalls

Confusing the lesion with acute osteoporotic vertebral compression fracture.

Selected References

Baur A, Stäbler A, Brüning R, et al. Diffusion-weighted MR imaging of bone marrow: differentiation of benign versus pathologic vertebral compression fractures. Radiology 1998; 207(2): 349–356

Cuénod CA, Laredo JD, Chevret S, et al. Acute vertebral collapse due to osteoporosis or malignancy: appearance on unenhanced and gadolinium-enhanced MR images. Radiology 1996; 199(2): 541–549

Fourney DR, Gokaslan ZL. Spinal instability and deformity due to neoplastic conditions [review]. Neurosurg Focus 2003; 14(1): e8

Taneichi H, Kaneda K, Takeda N, Abumi K, Satoh S. Risk factors and probability of vertebral body collapse in metastases of the spine. Spine 1997; 22(3): 239–245

Definition

▶ **Epidemiology**
Benign proliferation of normal or abnormal vascular components ● Most common soft-tissue tumor ● Most common tumor in early childhood and children (12%) ● 7% of all benign soft-tissue tumors ● Women more frequently affected.

▶ **Etiology, pathophysiology, pathogenesis**
Classified by predominant type of vessel seen histologically:
- Capillary hemangioma: consists entirely of capillaries ● Common form ● Often found in the skin and subcutaneous fatty tissue ● Spontaneous regression possible.
- Cavernous hemangioma: strongly dilated capillaries ● Deep soft tissues ● Less common ● No spontaneous regression ● Often calcified (up to 50%), resulting in phleboliths.
- Venous hemangioma: strong vessel walls with smooth muscle ● Commonly seen in children ● Mainly in upper half of body ● Slow blood flow ● Phleboliths possible.
- Arteriovenous hemangioma (arteriovenous malformation): abnormal communication between arteries and veins ● Arteriovenous shunts and resultant high blood flow possible.

Another classification divides vascular malformations into high-flow and low-flow lesions ● Typically superficial ● Deep structures such as skeletal muscle less commonly affected ● Synovial hemangiomas very rare (almost exclusively involving the knee) ● Several syndromes are associated with soft-tissue hemangiomas:
- Maffucci syndrome: multiple enchondromas and cavernous hemangiomas ● Especially affecting hands and feet ● Malignant transformation is possible.
- Klippel–Trénaunay–Weber syndrome: cutaneous hemangiomas ● Hypertrophy of bone and soft tissues ● Varicosis.
- Kasabach–Merritt syndrome: large hemangiomas ● Thrombocytopenia ● Purpura.

Imaging Signs

▶ **Modality of choice**
MRI ● MR angiography (MRA) ● Angiography for embolization.

▶ **Radiographic findings**
Soft-tissue swelling ● Round calcifications (phleboliths) or (less often) ossifications may be seen ● Osseous involvement is rare.

▶ **MRI findings**
T2-weighted images demonstrate lobulated formations with high signal intensity ("cluster of grapes" appearance) ● Vessels appear as dilated and tortuous structures ● Fluid–fluid levels may be seen within vessels composed of cystic spaces ● Punctate hypointense areas arising from fibrosis, faster flow ("flow voids"), or calcifications ● Thromboses appear as round, hypointense areas ● Typically intermediate signal (between muscle and fat) on T1-weighted images ● Peripheral fat sometimes present.

Fig. 1.37 a–c Extensive soft-tissue hemangioma involving the foot and ankle. MRI showing lobulated formations in the muscle and surrounding fatty and connective tissues.
a STIR image. Hyperintense signal.
b T1-weighted image. Signal isointense to muscle with isolated foci that are isointense to fat.

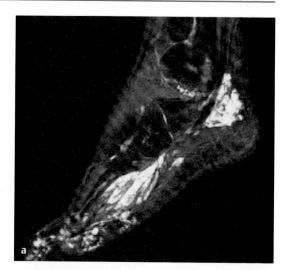

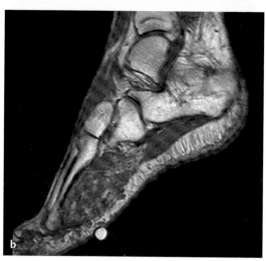

c T2-weighted image. Hyperintense signal.

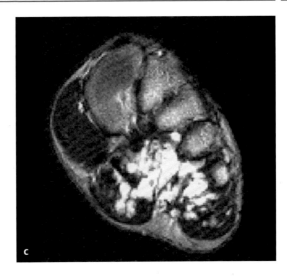

MRA: Distinguish high-flow and low-flow hemangiomas ● Distinguish arterial and venous vessels ● Capillary and cavernous hemangiomas demonstrate pooling after administration of contrast material ● Await late phase in venous hemangiomas.

Clinical Aspects

▶ **Typical presentation**
Soft-tissue swelling ● Palpable, sometimes pulsating lesions ● Pain ● Often an incidental finding ● Very large hemangiomas may lead to increased cardiac output as a result of arteriovenous shunting.

▶ **Treatment options**
Asymptomatic lesions do not require treatment given the frequency of spontaneous regression ● Generous excision to avoid recurrence (high hemorrhage risk) ● Embolization before excision or for inoperable high-flow hemangiomas ● Sclerotherapy for capillary and cavernous angiomas.

▶ **Course and prognosis**
Spontaneous involution common in children and adolescents ● Tendency to recur after incomplete excision.

▶ **What does the clinician want to know?**
Type of hemangioma ● Location and extent ● Can biopsy be avoided, given the high risk of hemorrhage?

Differential Diagnosis

Glomus tumor	– Usually subungual
Angiosarcoma, hemangiopericytoma, hemangioendothelioma	– Especially in older patients – Lymphedema – Calcifications are uncommon – No fat overgrowth
Hematoma	– Vessels cannot be discerned – No flow voids
Lymphangioma	– Affects lymphatic vessels, but not blood vessels – Often diffuse pattern of involvement with marked swelling – Frequently cystic: 95% neck or axilla – Manifestation by age 2 in 90%

Tips and Pitfalls

Low-flow hemangiomas usually cannot be depicted by angiography (arterial).

Selected References

Greenspan A, McGahan JP, Vogelsang P, Szabo RM. Imaging strategies in the evaluation of soft-tissue hemangiomas of the extremities: correlation of the findings of plain radiography, angiography, CT, MRI, and ultrasonography in 12 histologically proven cases. Skeletal Radiol 1992; 21(1): 11–18

Olsen K, Stacy G, Montag A. Soft tissue cavernous hemangiomas. Radiographics 2004; 24(3): 849–854

Resnick D, Kransdorf M. Bone and joint imaging. 3rd ed. Philadelphia: Elsevier, 2005: 718–719

Vilanova J, Barcelo J, Smirniotopoulos JG, et al. Hemangioma from head to toe: MR imaging with pathologic correlation [review]. Radiographics 2004; 24(2): 367–385

Definition
....

▶ **Epidemiology**
   Incidence of 1–2 : 100 000 ● 40% of patients are over age 40 ● Benign soft-tissue tumors are 100 times more common than malignant ones ● Male to female ratio 3:2.

▶ **Etiology, pathophysiology, pathogenesis**
   Heterogenous group of malignant mesenchymal tumors ● Location: 40% in lower extremity; 30% involving trunk; 15% involving head, throat, neck; 15% in upper extremity; seldom retroperitoneal ● Histology: leiomyosarcoma, fibrosarcoma, liposarcoma, rhabdomyosarcoma (mostly children), malignant fibrous histiocytoma (commonest malignant soft-tissue tumor in adults), neurogenic sarcoma, mesothelioma, rhabdomyosarcoma, hemangiosarcoma (very rare), synovial sarcoma ● Space-occupying lesion with displacement of local structures ● Formation of pseudocapsule ● High-risk sarcomas: > 5 cm, deep in muscle compartment, histological grade II–III.

Imaging Signs
....

▶ **Modality of choice**
   Local staging: MRI ● Staging of distant metastases: thoracic/abdominal CT.

▶ **Pathognomonic findings**
   Smoothly bordered soft-tissue mass involving the extremities.

▶ **Radiographic findings**
   Detection or exclusion of bony destruction.

▶ **MRI findings**
   Round, smoothly bordered soft-tissue mass (pseudocapsule) ● Location: superficial (subcutaneous) or deep (intramuscular), often on thigh ● Usually confined to one compartment ● Hypointense on T1-weighted SE images ● Hyperintense on T2-weighted SE images ● Peritumoral edema commonly found ● Diffuse enhancement after contrast administration ● Central area of necrosis may be found, especially in rapidly growing tumors.
   Liposarcoma: Fatty elements within the tumor ● Usually has areas with a feathery appearance and signal intensity equal to that of fat on T1-weighted SE images ● Highly differentiated liposarcomas show less enhancement after administration of contrast material than dedifferentiated tumors ● Myxoid tumor components and necrosis appear hyperintense on T2-weighted SE images.
   Synovial sarcoma: Para-articular location ● Septations and fluid-fluid levels due to hemorrhage ● Calcifications typically detected (on radiography and CT).

Fig. 1.38 A 67-year-old man with syno-vial sarcoma in the left gluteal muscles. Radiograph demonstrating typical calcifi-cations within the tumor.

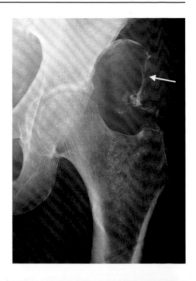

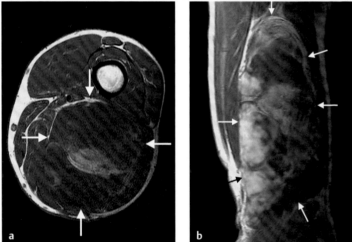

Fig. 1.39 a, b A 36-year-old man with liposarcoma in the flexor compartment of the left thigh.

a Axial T1-weighted SE sequence. Hypointense tumor with typical hyperintense septal components indicative of its lipoid origin.

b The tumor demonstrates marked contrast enhancement.

Clinical Aspects

▶ **Typical presentation**
Primary symptom: painless swelling ● In 20–30% of cases local or referred pain ● Generalized signs of tumor (weight loss, weakness, anemia).

▶ **Treatment options**
Treatment depends on tumor stage and prognostic factors ● Compartment resection ● Preoperative and postoperative adjuvant chemotherapy, with or without regional hyperthermia, for high-risk sarcomas ● Postoperative radiation therapy, especially after R1/R2 resection.

▶ **Course and prognosis**
Hematogenous metastasis: lung (70%) ● Liver metastasis from abdominal and retroperitoneal primary tumors ● Lymphatic metastasis is rare ● Prognosis depends on histological grade, tumor size, extent and location ● Low-grade tumors (grade I) carry a 5-year survival rate of 75%; intermediate-grade, differentiated tumors 56%; high-grade (grade III) tumors 26% ● High rate of local recurrence of liposarcoma and malignant fibrous histiocytoma (up to 45%).

▶ **What does the clinician want to know?**
Location of tumor: superficial or deep in muscle compartment ● Tumor size and extent ● Invasion of vessels, nerves, or bones ● Distant metastasis?

Differential Diagnosis

Lipoma	– Differentiate from liposarcoma – T1-weighted images show only fatty tissue with hyperintense signal – No hyperintense components on fat-saturated images – Nonenhancing after contrast administration – No calcification
Hematoma	– No solid components – Only peripheral contrast enhancement – Patient history
Extraosseous bone tumors	– E.g., Ewing sarcoma: impossible to distinguish
Myositis ossificans	– Patient history: trauma – At 7–10 days, soft-tissue swelling – At 2–6 weeks, calcification – At 6–8 weeks, ossification

Tips and Pitfalls

Mistaking the lesion for a benign soft-tissue tumor or hematoma.

Selected References

Varma DG. Optimal radiologic imaging of soft tissue sarcomas. Semin Surg Oncol 1999; 17(1): 2–10

Hanna SL, Fletcher BD. MR imaging of malignant soft-tissue sarcomas. Magn Reson Imaging Clin N Am 1995; 3(4): 629–640

Cormier JN, Pollock RE. Soft tissue sarcomas. CA Cancer J Clin 2004; 54(2): 94–109

Goldberg BR. Soft tissue sarcoma: an overview [review]. Orthop Nurs 2007; 26(1): 4–11; quiz 12–13

Sim FH, Edmonson JH, Wold LE. Soft-tissue sarcomas. Future perspectives [review]. Clin Orthop Relat Res 1993; (289): 106–112

Pappo AS, Parham DM, Rao BN, Lobe TE. Soft tissue sarcomas in children [review]. Semin Surg Oncol 1999; 16(2): 121–143

Definition

▶ **Epidemiology**
Most common benign soft-tissue tumor • Age predilection: 30–50 years •
Women more often affected than men.

▶ **Etiology, pathophysiology, pathogenesis**
Benign tumor of adipose tissue (histology reveals exclusively mature fatty tissue
without atypical cells) • Fibrous capsule • Partly permeated by fibrous tissue
septae • Intraosseous lipomas are rare • Variants: myolipoma, angiolipoma.
Location: superficial (subcutaneous) or deep (intrafascial, intramuscular) •
Predilection for shoulder, back, extremities.

Imaging Signs

▶ **Modality of choice**
MRI.

▶ **Radiographic findings**
Usually not recognizable • Calcifications possible • Can cause cortical thickening
or erosion if located near bone.

▶ **Ultrasound**
Usually smooth-bordered, hyperechoic mass • Calcifications give hyperechoic
signal within the mass with acoustic shadows.

▶ **CT findings**
Homogeneous structure with density equal to adipose tissue (–50 to –100 HU) •
Smooth borders • Fluffy calcifications often found • Nonenhancing.

▶ **MRI findings**
Signal intensity on all sequences similar to that of subcutaneous adipose tissue •
Hyperintense on T1-weighted SE images • Hyperintense on T2-weighted SE images • Homogeneous signal, permeated in parts by thin, hypointense connective
tissue septa • No intratumoral or septal enhancement after contrast administration.

Clinical Aspects

▶ **Typical presentation**
Nonspecific symptoms • Soft, palpable nodule or swelling • Very slow growth.

▶ **Treatment options**
Treatment is generally unnecessary • For larger tumors or suspected liposarcoma, excision with capsule.

▶ **Course and prognosis**
Very good, since the tumor is benign.

▶ **What does the clinician want to know?**
Extent • Neurovascular compression • Rule out liposarcoma.

Tumors

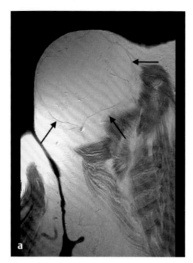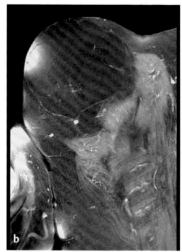

Fig. 1.40 a, b A 75-year-old woman with a large, subcutaneous lipoma behind the shoulder.
a Coronal T1-weighted SE sequence. Large mass with septa and isointense to fat.
b Postcontrast fat-saturated T1-weighted SE sequence. No intratumoral or septal enhancement, so liposarcoma can be ruled out.

Differential Diagnosis

Liposarcoma	– Enhances after contrast administration; in grade I lesions septa may enhance only minimally
	– Marked contrast enhancement in grade II and III lesions
Angiolipoma	– Vascular loops within tumor
	– Enhancement after contrast administration

Tips and Pitfalls

Mistaking the lesion for liposarcoma.

Selected References

Campbell RS, Grainger AJ, Mangham DC, Beggs I, Teh J, Davies AM. Intraosseous lipoma: report of 35 new cases and a review of the literature. Skeletal Radiol 2003; 32(4): 209–222

Kransdorf MJ, Bancroft LW, Peterson JJ, Murphey MD, Foster WC, Temple HT. Imaging of fatty tumors: distinction of lipoma and well-differentiated liposarcoma. Radiology 2002; 224(1): 99–104

Murphey MD, Carroll JF, Flemming DJ, Pope TL, Gannon FH, Kransdorf MJ. From the archives of the AFIP: benign musculoskeletal lipomatous lesions [review]. Radiographics 2004; 24(5): 1433–1466

Woertler K. Soft tissue masses in the foot and ankle: characteristics on MR imaging. Semin Musculoskelet Radiol 2005; 9(3): 227–242

Definition

Synonyms: synovial endothelioma, giant cell tumor of tendon sheaths

▶ **Epidemiology**

Age predilection: 20–40 years ● Intra-articular variant is most common tumor-like process affecting a joint ● Giant cell tumor of tendon sheath is the most common soft-tissue tumor of the hand ● Any joint may be involved, especially those in the extremities.

▶ **Etiology, pathophysiology, pathogenesis**

Benign lesion ● Considered to be a tumor-like, soft-tissue lesion ● Lesions may be intra-articular or in bursae and tendon sheaths (giant-cell tumor of tendon sheath) ● Villous proliferation of synovial tissue ● Contains hemosiderin ● May destroy adjacent bone ● Growth diffuse or localized.

Imaging Signs

▶ **Modality of choice**

MRI ● Radiography.

▶ **Pathognomonic findings**

Soft-tissue tumor in a joint or along tendon sheath with hemosiderin deposits.

▶ **Radiographic/CT findings**

Soft-tissue mass ● High density (hemosiderin deposits) ● No calcifications ● No narrowing of joint space ● When there is bone involvement (30–40%), well-defined osteolytic lesions near the joint, usually with a sclerotic rim.

▶ **MRI findings**

Nodular soft-tissue mass ● Most commonly involves the knee joint (60–80%) ● Less often found along tendon sheaths in the hands or feet ● Hypointense on T1-weighted images ● Hypointense on T2-weighted TSE images ● Diffuse enhancement after administration of contrast material ● Diagnostic clues include location in joint, bursa, or along tendon sheath, and presence of hemosiderin deposits ● Hemosiderin appears as a signal void on susceptibility-sensitive sequences (T2*-weighted gradient-echo images).

Clinical Aspects

▶ **Typical presentation**

Intermittent swelling and pain about the affected joint ● Joint stiffness occasionally.

▶ **Treatment options**

PVNS of the tendon sheath and bursae: resection ● PVNS of the joint: open synovectomy, perhaps with additional radiation synovectomy.

▶ **Course and prognosis**

Curable, but high rate of recurrence.

▶ **What does the clinician want to know?**

Extent ● Osseous involvement ● Rule out synovial sarcoma.

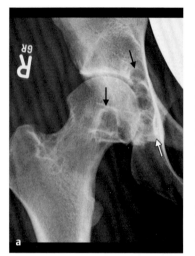 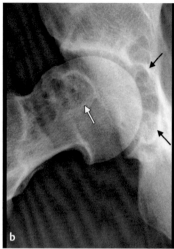

Fig. 1.41 a, b   A 31-year-old woman with gradually worsening pain in the right hip joint. Radiographs of the hip joint in two planes. PVNS of the hip with multiple, sharply defined osteolyses with sclerotic rim in the acetabulum and femoral neck.

Fig. 1.42   A 43-year-old man. MRI of right knee joint. T2-weighted image showing intra-articular PVNS as a well-circumscribed, hypointense, nodular soft-tissue formation in the Hoffa's fat pad.

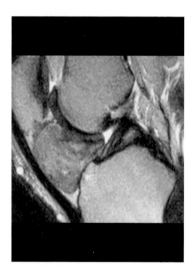

Differential Diagnosis

Synovial sarcoma	– Calcifications within tumor
	– No osseous lesions on either side of the joint
	– Poorly defined erosion of bone (always biopsy!)
Arthritis	– Symmetrical narrowing of joint space
	– No soft-tissue tumors
Joint deterioration	– Localized narrowing of joint space
	– No soft-tissue tumors
Intraosseous ganglion	– Confined to the bone (epiphysis)
	– Signal intensity on MRI typical of cystic formations
	– No soft-tissue tumor

Tips and Pitfalls

Failure to obtain T2*-weighted GE images to detect typical hemosiderin deposits •
Failure to obtain radiographs to rule out calcifications, which are indicative of malignancy (synovial sarcoma).

Selected References

Al-Nakshabandi NA, Ryan AG, Choudur H, et al. Pigmented villonodular synovitis. Clin Radiol 2004; 59(5): 414–420

Bravo SM, Winalski CS, Weissman BN. Pigmented villonodular synovitis [review]. Radiol Clin North Am 1996; 34(2): 311–326, x–xi

Cheng XG, You YH, Liu W, Zhao T, Qu H. MRI features of pigmented villonodular synovitis. Clin Rheumatol 2004; 23(1): 31–34

Masih S, Antebi A. Imaging of pigmented villonodular synovitis [review]. Semin Musculoskelet Radiol 2003; 7(3): 205–216

Definition

▶ **Epidemiology and classification**

Myositis ossificans circumscripta (localisata):
- Post-traumatic: Age predilection is usually before 30 years • Men are more often affected than women.
- No history of trauma • neuropathic form: especially in head trauma or paraplegia (20–25%), no sex predilection • Idiopathic form.

Myositis ossificans progressiva (Münchmeyer disease): Less than 600 cases in the literature.

▶ **Etiology, pathophysiology, pathogenesis**

Extraosseous, nonneoplastic new bone formation.

Post-traumatic myositis ossificans circumscripta: Associated with traumatic muscle or soft-tissue injury • Predilection for proximal regions of the extremities and the hip region • Often a postoperative event • More than 60% of cases occur after total hip arthroplasty • Relevant symptoms in 10–20% of cases • Joint stiffness in 10%.

Neuropathic myositis ossificans circumscripta: Associated with paraplegia or head trauma • At shoulder or elbow joint (after head trauma) or distal to spinal cord injury • Etiology unclear • Neurodegenerative and inflammatory mechanisms possible.

Myositis ossificans progressiva: Congenital, hereditary form (very rare) • Usually new mutation • Some evidence of autosomal dominant inheritance • Ossifications in muscle, tendons, aponeuroses, and skin.

Imaging Signs

▶ **Modality of choice**

Radiography • CT.

▶ **Radiographic findings**

At least 3–4 weeks after trauma, indistinct, cloudy densities appear in soft tissue • After 6–8 weeks, a peripheral margin of cortical bone is clearly distinguishable • Ossification progresses from the periphery towards the center • The center generally remains free of ossified tissue • The lesion is usually separate from adjacent skeletal elements.

Neuropathic myositis ossificans circumscripta: Usually extensive calcifications about the elbow and shoulder joints or, in paraplegic patients, distal to site of spinal cord injury • Lesions may resemble those in the post-traumatic form or may be arranged linearly along muscle fibers.

Myositis ossificans progressiva: Spreads from cranial to caudal and from dorsal to ventral • Central ossification possible • Multilocular.

▶ **CT findings**

Zonal pattern (calcified peripheral zone with uncalcified center) is better depicted than on radiographs • Distance from adjacent bone cortex is also visualized better.

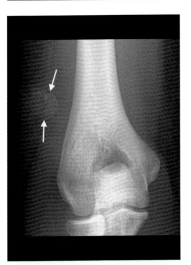

Fig. 1.43 A 29-year-old man with pain in the right upper arm and a 2-month history of difficulty in extending the joint. No remembered trauma. Elbow radiograph. Smooth-bordered, round ossification in the soft tissues lateral to the distal humerus. Myositis ossificans confirmed on biopsy.

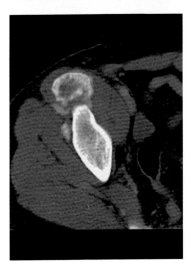

Fig. 1.44 A 32-year-old man. CT scan. Trauma involving the right inguinal region several years before presentation. At the attachment site of the rectus femoris is a round, mature ossification with peripheral neocortical formation, typical of myositis ossificans. Unlike parosteal osteosarcoma, in myositis ossificans calcification is greater at the periphery than at the center.

▶ **MRI findings**

Localized space-occupying mass ● Hyperintense in some parts, hypointense in others (areas of hemorrhage) on T2-weighted images ● Usually hypointense on T1-weighted images (hyperintense in parts if recent hemorrhage) ● Often surrounded by soft-tissue or muscle edema ● Inhomogeneous contrast enhancement ● Sometimes ring-like contrast enhancement ● Central zone more readily distinguished in more mature lesions: on T2-weighted and STIR images there is inhomogeneous, intermediate to high signal intensity ● Peripheral areas of signal loss (ossifications) on T1-weighted and T2-weighted images.

▶ **Nuclear medicine**

Markedly increased uptake of ^{99m}Tc on bone scans ● Good marker for activity of disease process ● Low specificity ● Rules out multifocal lesions (myositis ossificans progressiva, battered child syndrome).

Clinical Aspects

▶ **Typical presentation**

Post-traumatic form: Pain is initially progressive, then subsides again after 2–3 months ● Usually involves thigh, buttocks, and elbow ● Especially in neuropathic form, massive joint-bridging ossifications ● Joint stiffness possible.

Myositis ossificans progressiva: Multiple, predominantly periarticular ossifications that may lead to complete immobilization ● Laboratory tests for evaluating disease course: serum alkaline phosphatase levels (correlate well with disease activity, as does scintigraphy).

▶ **Treatment options**

In post-traumatic form initial treatment is conservative (local cooling in acute phase, NSAIDs, bisphosphonates) ● Surgical removal is an option after bone formation has ceased ● Treatment goal: to re-establish joint functioning.

▶ **Course and prognosis**

Spontaneous resolution possible (but rare) in post-traumatic form ● In myositis ossificans progressiva, progressive loss of mobility starts early, even during early adulthood ● Death is usually from infection (pneumonia).

▶ **What does the clinician want to know?**

Extent ● Full extent of disease process ● Distinguish from tumors (especially osteosarcoma).

Differential Diagnosis

Osteosarcoma	– Ossification usually more marked in the center of the lesion than peripherally
	– Arises from bone; in parosteal osteosarcoma, usually rests directly on the cortex
	– Generally no history of trauma as in myositis ossificans

Tips and Pitfalls

Mistaking myositis ossificans for osteosarcoma.

Selected References

Armfield DR, Kim DH, Towers JD, Bradley JP, Robertson DD. Sports-related muscle injury in the lower extremity [review]. Clin Sports Med 2006; 25(4): 803–842

Elsayes KM, Lammle M, Shariff A, Totty WG, Habib IF, Rubin DA. Value of magnetic resonance imaging in muscle trauma [review]. Curr Probl Diagn Radiol 2006; 35(5): 206–212

McCarthy EF, Sundaram M. Heterotopic ossification: a review. Skeletal Radiol 2005; 34(10): 609–619

Parikh J, Hyare H, Saifuddin A. The imaging features of post-traumatic myositis ossificans, with emphasis on MRI [review]. Clin Radiol 2002; 57(12): 1058–1066

Park KS, Kang SG, Cho CS, Kim HY. Clinical images: myositis ossificans of the upper extremity. Arthritis Rheum 2007; 56(7): 2454

Definition

▶ **Epidemiology**
Infection of the bone and bone marrow • Incidence of hematogenous osteomyelitis is decreasing worldwide and is very low in industrialized nations • Postoperative and post-traumatic osteomyelitis are increasing • Usually affects metaphyses of long tubular bones.

▶ **Etiology, pathophysiology, pathogenesis**
Classification:
– Acute osteomyelitis.
– Chronic (> 6 weeks) and subacute (see Brodie abscess).
– Post-traumatic and postoperative osteomyelitis.
– Special variant: chronic recurrent multifocal osteomyelitis (CRMO) • Chronic, systemic, aseptic inflammation of uncertain etiology • Multifocal • Prolonged course (2–5% of all osteomyelitis infections) • More common among children and adolescents.

Classification by pathogenesis:
– Hematogenous infection (e.g., in otitis, angina).
– Infection spread by extension from adjacent tissues (e.g., urogenital infection).
– Direct bacterial inoculation (penetrating injury, puncture, operation).

Usually triggered by a single pathogen (e.g., *Staphylococcus aureus* in 30%; in children often caused by *Haemophilus influenzae*) • Critical bacterial count for infection decreases dramatically (by several orders of magnitude) if foreign material is present (e.g., total endoprosthesis, osteosynthesis material).

Risk factors: (open) fractures, foreign material, suppressed immunocompetence (cancer, diabetes mellitus, arterial occlusive disease, immunosuppressants), indwelling vascular access devices, drug abuse • Abscesses, sequestra, and cloacae are the starting point (as well as imaging signs) of chronicity.

Imaging Signs

▶ **Modality of choice**
Radiography • MRI.

▶ **Radiographic findings**
Acute osteomyelitis: Unremarkable findings up to 14 days after symptom onset • Soft-tissue swelling (beginning on 3rd–5th day) • Osteoporosis (after 1 week and only detectable after about 30% loss of bone density) • Irregular area of osteolysis with indistinct border and no surrounding sclerosis (after 2–3 weeks) • In children, periosteal (usually lamellated) reaction possible after only 5 days • Sequestration after 3–6 weeks.
Chronic osteomyelitis: Mixed picture of bone destruction and sclerosis • Sequestra • Involucrum (sequestral cavity) • Sinus tracts • Active infection indicated by new areas of bone lysis and periosteal reaction • Position and extent of (often communicating) sinus tracts can be visualized by contrast filling on radiography.

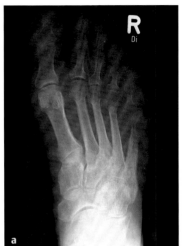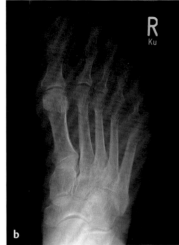

Fig. 2.1 a, b   Radiographic images of acute osteomyelitis in a patient with diabetes mellitus.

a Ill-defined osteolytic destruction of the distal portion of the fifth metatarsal shaft and the MTP joint. Marked osteopenia and subtle periosteal reaction.

b Radiograph from 3 weeks earlier shows only soft-tissue swelling.

▶ **CT findings**

Modality of choice for detailed assessment of bone destruction and sequestration ● CT-guided biopsy to obtain bacterial sample ● Drainage device.

▶ **MRI findings**

Potential for early and certain diagnosis ● Exact evaluation of intraosseous and extraosseous involvement ● The most sensitive studies are STIR, fat-saturated proton-density-weighted, and T1-weighted sequences after administration of contrast material ● These sequences (unlike noncontrast T1-weighted sequences) have a tendency, however, to overestimate extent of involvement ● Abscesses and sinus tracts are directly visualized by enhancing sinus wall or abscess membrane on postcontrast fat-saturated T1-weighted sequences read in conjunction with the high signal intensity of fluid accumulation on fat-saturated T2-weighted and STIR sequences ● Extensive perifocal edema often present.

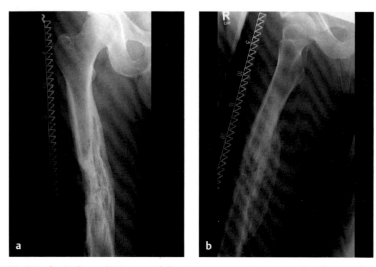

Fig. 2.2 a, b Radiographic images of chronic post-traumatic osteomyelitis diagnosed in the patient 10 years earlier. Extensive periosteal and endosteal sclerosis alternating with radiolucencies, some with indistinct borders.

Clinical Aspects

▶ **Typical presentation**
   Acute osteomyelitis: Area of warmth, redness, and pain • Swelling • Sinus tract leading to surface • Restricted mobility • Fever • Increased inflammatory parameters.
   Chronic osteomyelitis: Often little evidence of infection on laboratory tests or in terms of generalized and local signs • Often protracted course persisting for decades with intermittent periods of disease inactivity.
▶ **Treatment options**
   Surgical debridement • Systemic and local antibiotics.
▶ **Course and prognosis**
   Early diagnosis is essential to avoid chronicity.
▶ **What does the clinician want to know?**
   Confirm diagnosis • Location and extent of bone and soft-tissue involvement • Assess activity (reactivation of chronic osteomyelitis?) • Treatment progress • Rule out differential diagnoses (especially malignant bone tumors).

Differential Diagnosis

Bone tumors (e.g., Ewing sarcoma, osteosarcoma, eosinophilic granuloma), metastases	– Patient history and examination (diabetes, ulcer?), perhaps laboratory studies – Periosteal reaction often, but not always, more aggressive in Ewing sarcoma (Codman triangle, "sunburst" appearance) – Biopsy if diagnosis uncertain
Traumatic lesions, stress fracture	– Patient history – Fracture line
Post-traumatic changes	– Patient history – Contrast studies not useful until at least 9 months after surgery

Tips and Pitfalls

Osteomyelitis cannot be ruled out on the basis of negative radiographic findings alone • In a patient with known soft-tissue infection, the appearance of a new area of osseous destruction, as well as abscess or sequestra formation, are evidence of osteomyelitis.

Selected References

Calhoun JH, Manring MM. Adult osteomyelitis. Infect Dis Clin North Am 2005; 19(4): 765–786

Chatha DS, Cunningham PM, Schweitzer ME. MR imaging of the diabetic foot: diagnostic challenges. Radiol Clin North Am 2005l; 43(4): 747–759, ix

Lazzarini L, Mader JT, Calhoun JH. Osteomyelitis in long bones. J Bone Joint Surg Am 2004; 86-A(10): 2305–2318

Offiah AC. Acute osteomyelitis, septic arthritis and diskitis: differences between neonates and older children. Eur J Radiol 2006; 60(2): 221–232

Definition

▶ **Epidemiology**
Rare form of subacute or primary chronic osteomyelitis ● Typically affects children and adolescents ● 3–5% of all osteomyelitis infections ● 40% manifest in 2nd decade ● Boys more often affected than girls.

▶ **Etiology, pathophysiology, pathogenesis**
Subacute form of osteomyelitis with circumscribed foci ● Usually caused by hematogenous spread of staphylococcal bacteria ● Pathognomonic findings include a ring-shaped border around the focus of infection in the bone marrow (granulation tissue).

Imaging Signs

▶ **Modality of choice**
Radiography ● MRI.

▶ **Radiographic findings**
Typically elongated lesion presenting as an area of increased radiolucency with a distinct border ● Margin of reactive sclerosis ● Sequestra rarely detected (20%) ● There may be a typically radiolucent sinus tract from abscess to epiphyseal plate ● In 40–50% of cases periosteal bone apposition and cortical thickening are seen ● Lesions are single or multiple ● May cross the growth plate ● Usually 1–5 cm in size ● Most common location: tibial metaphysis, followed by femoral metaphysis ● Transgression of epiphysis is rare (occurs mostly in young children) ● Diaphyseal lesions present in 30%.

▶ **CT findings**
Visualization of gas foci, sequestra, sinus tracts ● Method of choice for demonstrating osseous destruction and to guide biopsy.

▶ **MRI findings**
Better visualization of extent (growth plate involvement) ● Detection of renewed activity ● Circumscribed lesion, the center of which is hypointense on T1-weighted images and hyperintense on T2-weighted and STIR images ● Inner abscess wall is isointense to muscle on T1-weighted images ● Outer abscess wall is usually relatively wide and hypointense on all sequences ● Rarely, a peripheral halo sign is seen (hypointense on T1-weighted images) ● After administration of contrast material, center of lesion is nonenhancing (representing necrosis) and abscess wall enhances ● Peripheral edema may be seen in the bone marrow and paraosseous soft tissues ● Extent appears to correlate with acuteness of infection.

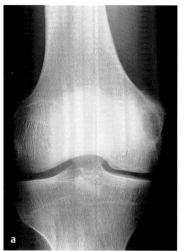

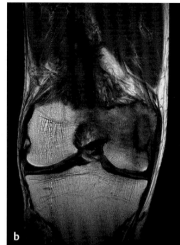

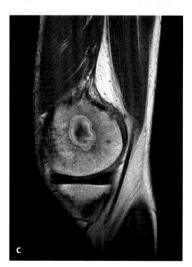

Fig. 2.3 a–c Brodie abscess in a 20-year-old man with a long-standing history of intermittent periods of swelling, local warmth, and redness about the knee. No systemic signs of inflammation.
a Radiograph showing osteolytic destruction on the metaphysis with surrounding sclerosis and periosteal reaction.
b Coronal MRI, T1-weighted image. Confluent area typical of an abscess.
c Sagittal MRI, postcontrast T1-weighted image. Rim enhancement and perifocal edema.

Clinical Aspects

▶ **Typical presentation**
Onset is often insidious ● Generalized signs and symptoms often minimal or absent ● Often circumscribed swelling that is tender to palpation ● Laboratory results appear normal (in contrast to acute osteomyelitis).

▶ **Treatment options**
Curettage ● Surgical debridement ● Antibiotics.

▶ **Course and prognosis**
No risk of recurrence after complete surgical removal.

▶ **What does the clinician want to know?**
Location and extent ● Number (single or multiple lesions) ● Communication with epiphysis.

Differential Diagnosis

Eosinophilic granuloma	– Often no surrounding sclerosis
	– No confluent areas
Osteoid osteoma	– Typical nidus
	– Usually smaller than 1 cm
Traumatic lesion	– Less well-defined
	– Patient history
Aneurysmal bone cyst	– Often multilocular
	– Less extensive surrounding sclerosis
	– Fluid–fluid levels
	– Gradually increases in size
Other bone tumors	– Solid lesions

Tips and Pitfalls

Mistaking a lytic lesion for a bone tumor.

Selected References

Guermazi A, Mohr A, Genant H. Brodie abscess: another type of chronic posttraumatic osteomyelitis. Eur Radiol 2003; 13(7): 1750–1752

Martí-Bonmatí L, Aparisi F, Poyatos C, Vilar J. Brodie abscess: MR appearance in 10 patients. J Magn Reson Imaging 1993; 3(3): 543–546

Resnick D, Kransdorf M. Bone and joint imaging. 3rd ed. Philadelphia: Elsevier, 2005: 718–719

Inflammatory Diseases

Definition

▶ **Epidemiology**
Affects 2% of the population ● Peak incidence (diagnosis) in 4th and 5th decades ● Women affected 3–4 times more often than men ● Increased familial incidence ● Up to 70% of patients have HLA antigen DR4.

▶ **Etiology, pathophysiology, pathogenesis**
Chronic inflammatory disease ● Predilection for synovial membrane ● With disease progression, osseous destruction of affected joints ● Etiology is complex and incompletely understood ● Cellular immune reaction to an as yet unidentified antigen ● Synovium is the primary target organ of various immunological cascades, responding with inflammatory proliferative changes (pannus) ● Secondary destruction of the capsule–ligament complex, cartilage, and bone.

Imaging Signs

▶ **Modality of choice**
Radiography ● MRI.

▶ **Radiographic findings**
No radiologically identifiable skeletal changes in early disease ● Often bilateral, symmetrical, and usually polyarticular pattern of involvement ● Sites of predilection: phalangeal finger and toe joints as well as wrists ● Findings divided into three groups based on Dihlmann:
  – Soft-tissue swelling ● Joint effusion ● Synovitis
  – Collateral phenomenon in rheumatoid arthritis: band-like areas of juxta-articular osteoporosis
  – Direct signs: joint space widening (mainly due to joint effusion) ● Symmetrical narrowing of joint space is an indirect sign of joint destruction (especially marked between carpal bones) ● Erosions, sites of predilection: hand (MCP joints II–V, PIP, carpal bones, ulnar styloid process), foot (MTP joints II–V, IPJ) ● Early visualization of disrupted subchondral bone end plate ● Subchondral cysts ● Ulnar deviation of the fingers ● Buttonhole deformity and swan-neck deformity of the fingers ● Ankylosis as end-stage finding.
In cervical spine involvement, stepladder deformity, atlantoaxial dislocation, and pseudobasilar invagination.

▶ **MRI findings**
Symmetrical pattern of involvement is characteristic (see radiographic findings; DD: degenerative changes, psoriatic arthritis, gout) ● Detection of synovitis on contrast-enhanced images enables early diagnosis, estimate of disease activity, and early medication, if possible before onset of bone destruction ● Signal alterations analogous to those of bone marrow edema (especially on fat-saturated T2-weighted sequences) that have no corresponding findings in conventional radiographs represent pre-erosive changes, still potentially reversible ● Tendon sheath inflammation seen as increased signal intensity on T2-weighted images ● Direct imaging of cartilage destruction ● Dynamic contrast-enhanced sequences with rapid imaging time (less than 10 seconds per data set) appear to reflect

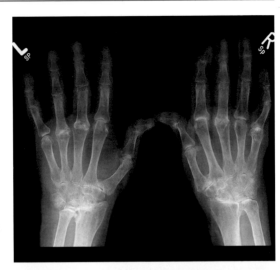

Fig. 2.4 Long-standing rheumatoid arthritis. Radiograph of both hands. Generalized osteopenia. Symmetrical pattern affecting the carpus, MCP joints, and (slight) involvement of the PIP joints. Complete joint destruction at some sites, but only joint narrowing at others. Secondary degenerative changes. Decreased carpal height on the left side and ulnar translocation of the carpus.

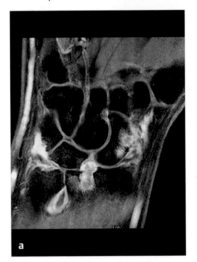

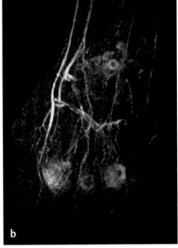

Fig. 2.5 a, b Rheumatoid arthritis. MRI.
a Fat-saturated T1-weighted SE sequence after administration of contrast material. Synovial enhancement in the carpus as well as radiocarpal and distal radioulnar joint. Involvement of scapholunate ligament and osseous erosion of the scaphoid.
b Dynamic, contrast-enhanced MIP in another patient. Early arterial contrast enhancement around MCP joints II–IV and wrist joints, indicative of florid inflammation.

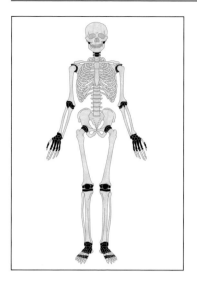

Fig. 2.6 Pattern of involvement in rheumatoid arthritis.

disease activity in terms of inflammatory changes involving the synovial membranes.

▶ **Nuclear medicine**
Three-phase bone scan ● Overview of pattern of involvement ● May provide evidence of disease when radiographic findings are negative.

▶ **Ultrasound findings**
Pannus (synovial proliferation, hyperechoic) ● Joint effusion ● Depiction of tendon sheaths (potential for targeted injection of antiphlogistic drugs) ● Baker cysts ● Tendon ruptures ● Power Doppler imaging: perfusion assessment (synovial hyperemia as indicator of disease activity).

Clinical Aspects
....

▶ **Typical presentation**
Nonspecific generalized symptoms ● Painfully swollen joints with limited mobility (Gaenslen sign: pain on pressure) ● Rheumatoid nodules ● In later stages, severe malalignment, subluxation, and fibrous ankylosis ● Periods of exacerbation and remission are typical ● Rarely, severe generalized signs of disease, fever, or extra-articular involvement occur.

▶ **Treatment options**
– Active and passive physical therapy (thermotherapy, cryotherapy, exercise therapy, massage therapy, physiotherapy).
– Medication (NSAIDs, glucocorticoids, disease-modifying drugs, and biologicals, which are agents that interfere directly in the process of immunomodulation).

– Radiation synovectomy, synovectomy.
– Reconstructive surgery and prosthetic joint replacement.

▶ **Course and prognosis**
Unfavorable prognosis: polyarticular involvement, high rheumatoid factor titer, high CRP levels, high ESR ● In one-third of patients, joint changes lead to disability after a few years ● Life expectancy may be decreased by complications (e.g., secondary AA [reactive systemic] amyloidosis with nephrotic syndrome and possible renal insufficiency).

▶ **What does the clinician want to know?**
Stage and location ● Treatment monitoring (does joint destruction cease or continue to progress with treatment?).

Differential Diagnosis

Psoriasis	– Involvement of SI joint and entire spinal column – Enthesitis – Asymmetrical joint involvement more common – Coexisting proliferative and erosive changes
Reiter syndrome	– Asymmetrical oligoarthritis, especially of the lower extremities – Patient history: intestinal/urogenital infection – Usually unilateral SI joint involvement
Polyarthrosis/polyarthritis of the fingers	– Distal interphalangeal joints usually more severely affected than proximal; MCP joints not affected – No erosions except in erosive form of disease ("seagull sign")
Collagenosis	– Usually marked malalignment of wrist and finger joints, but no bony destruction

Tips and Pitfalls

Mistaking rheumatoid arthritis for one of the differential diagnoses.

Selected References

Keen HI, Brown AK, Wakefield RJ, Conaghan PG. MRI and musculoskeletal ultrasonography as diagnostic tools in early arthritis. Rheum Dis Clin North Am 2005; 31(4): 699–714

Sommer OJ, Kladosek A, Weiler V, et al. Rheumatoid arthritis: a practical guide to state-of-the-art imaging, image interpretation, and clinical implications. Radiographics 2005; 25(2): 381–398

Definition

▶ **Epidemiology**
Psoriasis: Disorder associated with genetic predisposition that affects the skin, mucous membranes, entheses, and joints • Polygenic multifactorial inheritance with threshold effect • Incidence in Europe: 2–3% • No sex predilection.
Psoriatic arthritis: Affects 5–7% of all psoriasis patients • Mostly occurs in type I psoriasis with increased familial incidence and early age of manifestation (10–25 years) • Frequently associated with HLA-B27 • Negative for rheumatoid factor.

▶ **Etiology, pathophysiology, pathogenesis**
Etiology unknown • Increased familial incidence of HLA antigens • Coexistence of erosive and proliferative bony changes • Increasing significance is attributed to enthesopathy.

Imaging Signs

▶ **Modality of choice**
Radiographs • MRI.

▶ **Radiographic findings**
Juxta-articular periosteal reaction in the form of subtle new bone formation (co-existence of periarticular bone proliferation and erosion results in "mouse ear" appearance) • Enthesopathy affecting the interphalangeal joints, calcaneus, ischial tuberosities, greater and lesser trochanters, malleoli, patella, olecranon, femoral condyles, and proximal tibia • Bone erosion begins in periarticular region • Later pencil-in-cup deformity • Periostitis along the diaphysis of long tubular bones • Soft-tissue swelling (involvement of entire digital ray leading to "sausage" fingers) • In patients with chronic sacroiliitis, co-existing erosive and sclerotic changes ("mixed picture", unilateral or bilateral involvement) • Chronic inflammatory changes affecting the corners of the vertebral bodies, which exhibit sclerosis ("shining corner" appearance) • Syndesmophytes • No or minimal juxta-articular osteoporosis.

▶ **CT findings**
Additional information about local severity of changes, especially in SI and temporomandibular joints and the sternum.

▶ **MRI findings**
Detection of early enthesopathy before appearance of bony changes • Periarticular findings: synovial inflammation (strongly enhancing), effusion • Sausage fingers: diffuse soft-tissue edema, perhaps tendon sheath inflammation • Distal phalanges of the fingers: edema, contrast enhancement of nail bed • Temporomandibular joint: slight anterior displacement of disk, condylar erosions, joint effusion.

Fig. 2.7 a–c
Psoriatic arthritis.
a Radiograph of right and left hands. Psoriatic arthritis of the MCP joint of the second finger of the left hand with marginal erosions, subtle new bone formation, and soft-tissue swelling. Erosions also at the MCP joint of the right thumb. Cortical thinning in the metadiaphyseal region of the middle phalanges of the left index finger and the right middle finger.

b Radiograph of right and left feet. Psoriatic arthritis involving all joints of the great toe as well as the MTP joints of the first through fourth toes with erosive changes, subtle new bone formation, and incipient lateral deviation. Erosive enthesopathy of the left navicular bone.

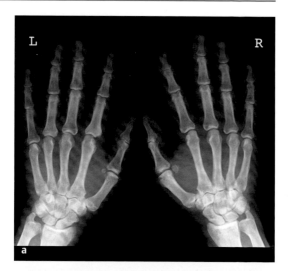

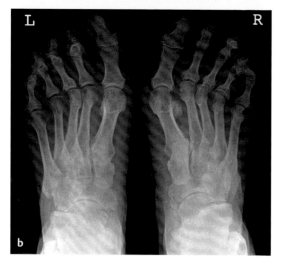

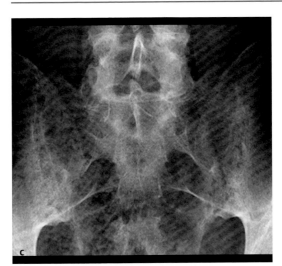

c Radiograph of SI joint. Asymmetrical, marked sacroiliac joint involvement with coexisting erosive and sclerotic changes.

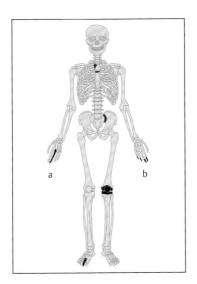

Fig. 2.8 a, b Pattern of involvement in psoriatic arthritis, with **a** whole-digital-ray involvement and **b** transverse involvement.

Clinical Aspects

▶ **Typical presentation**
Common patterns of involvement:
- Transverse involvement of DIP joints of the hands and feet.
- Involvement of all joints of a single digital ray ("sausage fingers").
- Asymmetrical oligoarthritis affecting large joints.
- Spondylitis.
- Sacroiliitis.

Joints are usually affected after initial skin changes ● In the more commonly occurring peripheral pattern of involvement, one or more smaller joints demonstrate acute, extremely painful, reddened areas of swelling ● Involvement of all joints of a finger ("sausage fingers") is typical. In the axial involvement pattern, additional stiffness of the sacroiliac joints and spinal column.

Clinical signs are divided into five subgroups of arthritic symptoms:
- Group 1: classic psoriatic arthritis ● Nail changes (erosion of tuberosities of distal phalanges: acro-osteolysis) ● DIP joints affected first, then PIP joints.
- Group 2: arthritis mutilans with "opera glass" hand deformity ● Extensive destruction of phalangeal and metacarpal joints ● Pencil-in-cup deformity ● Often involves other sites such as hip or elbow joints ● Sacroiliitis common.
- Group 3: symmetrical polyarthritis ● There may be ankylosis of DIP and PIP joints ● Often impossible to distinguish from rheumatoid arthritis.
- Group 4: asymmetrical oligoarthritis ● Involvement of DIP, PIP, and MCP joints.
- Group 5: spondylarthropathy with features resembling ankylosing spondylitis.

▶ **Treatment options**
Anti-inflammatory drugs are mainstay of treatment ● Local or systemic steroids ● Skin manifestations may be treated with, e.g., retinoids, psoralen and UVA light (PUVA) therapy, or TNF-α inhibitors.

▶ **Course and prognosis**
Disease occurs in episodes lasting months or years, often affecting different joints ● Joint function becomes restricted over the course of the disease ● Factors related to unfavorable prognosis: increased familial incidence, early onset (before age 20), polyarticular involvement, erosive changes, marked skin changes.

▶ **What does the clinician want to know?**
Assist diagnosis ● Extent of joint involvement.

Differential Diagnosis

Ankylosing spondylitis	– Usually bilateral SI joint involvement
(Bekhterev disease)	– Involvement of peripheral joints in background
Reiter syndrome	– Asymmetrical oligoarthritis, mainly involving lower extremities
	– Patient history: intestinal/urogenital infection
	– Usually unilateral SI joint involvement
Rheumatoid arthritis	– Symmetrical involvement of MCP or MTP joints
	– No enthesitis
Polyarthrosis/polyarthritis	– No skin lesions
of the fingers	– Difficult in a few cases

Tips and Pitfalls

Mistaking disease for a different type of arthropathy.

Selected References

Kane D, Pathare S. Early psoriatic arthritis. Rheum Dis Clin North Am 2005; 31(4): 641–657

Klecker RJ, Weissman BN. Imaging features of psoriatic arthritis and Reiter's syndrome. Semin Musculoskelet Radiol 2003; 7(2): 115–126

Ory PA, Gladman DD, Mease PJ. Psoriatic arthritis and imaging. Ann Rheum Dis 2005; 64(Suppl 2): ii55–ii57

Totterman SM. Magnetic resonance imaging of psoriatic arthritis: insight from traditional and three-dimensional analysis. Curr Rheumatol Rep 2004; 6(4): 317–321

Definition

▶ **Epidemiology**
Affects both sexes and all age groups equally ● Increased incidence among older, chronically ill patients, alcoholics, immunosuppressed individuals, drug addicts, and patients with pre-existing joint disease.

▶ **Etiology, pathophysiology, pathogenesis**
Most often iatrogenic (joint injection, surgery, trauma), due to spread of infection (e.g., in osteomyelitis), or hematogenous ● Infection of the joint can spread to the bone and lead to osteomyelitis ● Most common causative pathogen: staphylococci (60%) ● Other causative agents: pseudomonads, streptococci, gonococci, enterococci, and salmonellae ● Intra-articular release of chemotactic factors causes migration into the joint of polymorphonuclear leukocytes ● Lysosomal enzymes, collagenase, and cathepsin destroy the joint capsule ● Proliferation of synovial membrane (pannus) directly infiltrates and destroys the cartilage ● Fibrous or bony ankylosis may result if untreated.

Imaging Signs

▶ **Modality of choice**
Conventional radiography in two planes as primary study ● MRI.

▶ **Radiographic findings**
Early signs: soft-tissue swelling, effusion ● 10–14 days after onset of symptoms, periarticular osteoporosis due to inflammatory hyperemia ● Rapidly narrowing joint space as a result of cartilage destruction ● Erosion of bone, especially on "bare areas", caused by proliferating synovial membrane (pannus) ● Rapid joint destruction with disintegration of bony joint-bearing surfaces ● Joint malalignment.

▶ **MRI findings**
Early detection of joint effusion ● Abscesses may be seen ● Synovial contrast enhancement ● Often reactive bone marrow edema of involved joint structures (hypointense on T1-weighted images, hyperintense on fat-saturated images, enhancing after contrast administration) ● Accompanying osteomyelitis is difficult to distinguish from reactive marrow edema owing to similar signal intensity.

Clinical Aspects

▶ **Typical presentation**
Painfully restricted movement ● Severe joint pain ● Local warmth, redness, and swelling ● Low-grade fever, rarely chills ● Laboratory tests: inflammation markers, effusion culture positive.

▶ **Treatment options**
Systemic antibiotics ● Joint aspiration and cleansing ● In severe articular damage, joint replacement after healing of infection.

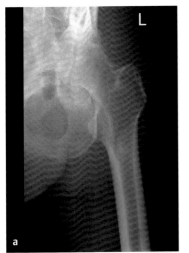
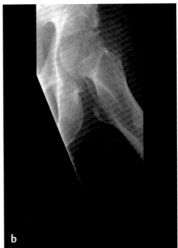

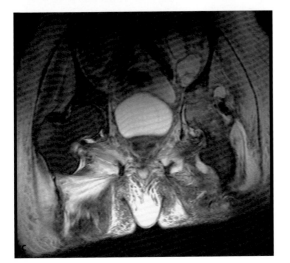

Fig. 2.9 a–c Septic arthritis in a 43-year-old man with a history of alcohol abuse and liver cirrhosis. Two-week history of pain in the left hip, intermittent fever, and high CRP levels.

a, b Radiographs of the left hip joint in two planes. Marked osteopenia around the joint, joint space narrowing, and incipient destruction of the femoral head.

c MRI. STIR sequence showing joint effusion, abscesses in the iliopsoas, and marrow edema in the femoral head and acetabulum.

▶ **Course and prognosis**

Often rapidly progressing ● Significant joint destruction ● Complications: sepsis, endocarditis, joint deterioration, fibrous or bony ankylosis, destruction of growth plate resulting in growth-related disorders or osteomyelitis.

▶ **What does the clinician want to know?**

Signs of inflammation ● Spread ● Effusion ● Joint destruction ● Cartilage destruction ● Rule out degenerative joint changes.

Differential Diagnosis

Degenerative joint changes	– Subchondral sclerosis, osteophytes, subchondral cysts
	– Active destructive process with bone marrow edema may resemble septic arthritis
	– Joint aspiration!
Rheumatoid arthritis	– Uniform narrowing of joint space
	– Signal cysts
	– Joint destruction occurs only in advanced long-standing disease (slow progression)
	– Pattern of involvement, patient history
PVNS	– Recurrent effusion
	– Cysts with sclerotic rim near the joint
	– Hemosiderin detectable on MRI

Tips and Pitfalls

Mistaking septic arthritis for degenerative joint disease—hence joint aspiration whenever septic arthritis is suspected!

Selected References

Resnick D, Kransdorf M. Osteomyelitis, septic arthritis and soft-tissue infection: mechanisms and situations. In: Bone and Joint Disorders. 4th ed. Phildelphia: Saunders, 2002: 2377–2481

Graif M, Schweitzer ME, Deely D, Mattencci T. The septic versus the nonseptic inflamed joint. Skeletal Radiol 1999; 28(11): 616–620

Greenspan A, Tehranzadeh J. Imaging of infectious arthritis. Radiol Clin North Am 2001; 39(2): 267–276

Learch TJ. Imaging of infectious arthritis [review]. Semin Musculoskelet Radiol 2003; 7(2): 137–142

Lee SK, Suh KJ, Kim YW, et al. Septic arthritis versus transient synovitis at MR imaging: preliminary assessment with signal intensity alterations in bone marrow. Radiology 1999; 211(2): 459–465

Definition

▶ **Epidemiology**
Crystal arthropathy with articular and extra-articular (e.g., kidney) urate crystal deposits • Manifests in 10% of patients with hyperuricemia (serum uric acid > 6.4 mg/dl, in 20–25% of male population, especially in wealthier nations) • Men are affected 20 times as often as women • Age of manifestation: after age 40 (in women, after menopause) • In 60%, disease affects the MTP joint of the great toe (podagra) • Also commonly affects the ankle, knee, and MCP joint of the thumb • In 40%, there is accompanying calcium pyrophosphate deposition disease (CPPD).

▶ **Etiology, pathophysiology, pathogenesis**
Imbalance between uric acid production and excretion • When serum concentrations exceed solubility limit, urate crystals precipitate in tissues • Leukocyte phagocytosis of urate crystals • Apoptosis with release of enzymes and mediators that cause damage to the joint.
Primary (familial) hyperuricemia: 90–95% • Enzyme defect affecting uric acid excretion or overproduction of uric acid • Poor diet.
Secondary hyperuricemia: Renal insufficiency • Diseases with accumulation of high levels of purine derivatives (myeloproliferative and lymphoproliferative disorders) • Cytostatic drugs and diuretics • Psoriasis • Endocrine disorders (e.g., hyperparathyroidism) • Alcohol.
Acute gout: Triggering factors include excessive drinking and dietary habits ("fasting and feasting") as well as stress.

Imaging Signs

▶ **Modality of choice**
Radiographs in two planes • Ultrasound • MRI.

▶ **Radiographic findings**
Early-stage or acute gout: Asymmetrical soft-tissue swelling near the joint.
Late-stage gout: 4- to 6-year latency in cases of inadequately treated gout • (Peri-)articular, well-defined erosions, often with sclerotic borders • Overhanging edges may be present without marked osteoporosis • Secondary degenerative joint changes in the course of disease • No juxta-articular osteopenia • Possibly accompanied by chondrocalcinosis.
Tophi: Inflammatory soft-tissue foci surrounding urate crystals • Calcification in renal damage • Spike-like tophi: spiculated periosteal reaction • Osseous tophi: well-defined, round osteolytic lesions with or without sclerotic rim.

▶ **Ultrasound findings**
Hyperechoic soft-tissue tophi • Central acoustic shadow representing centrally located crystal.

Fig. 2.10   Advanced gout. Radiograph of the hand showing marked tophaceous changes in the middle finger. Marginal erosions and soft-tissue swelling about the MCP joint of the index finger. A "spike" can be seen on the second metacarpal bone. Chondrocalcinosis in articular disk of distal radioulnar joint. Destruction also apparent in the distal radioulnar joint. Cystic destruction visible on the distal ulna.

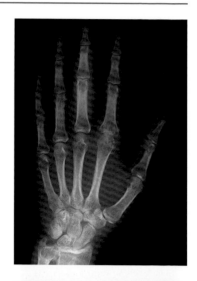

Fig. 2.11   Patient with known gout. Radiograph of the foot showing erosive changes on the medial aspect of the first metatarsal head overlapping the degenerative changes and indicating the presence of gout in addition to hallux valgus.

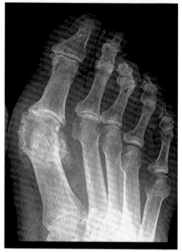

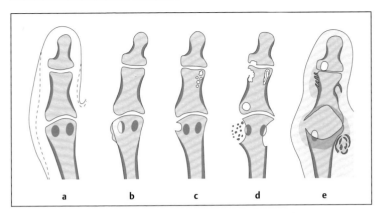

Fig. 2.12 a–e Typical findings affecting the great toe in a patient with gout.
a Soft-tissue swelling around the MTP joint related to gout (podagra).
b Radiolucency in the first metatarsal head caused by medullary tophus formation as well as discreet bone apposition on the medial aspect.
c Manifest erosion.
d Halberd-shaped appearance with expanding tophus.
e Marked tophaceous destruction of the MTP joint with saucer-like flattening of the articular surfaces and spike-like tophi on the proximal phalanx.

▶ **MRI findings**
In patients with unknown underlying disease, obtain MRI to rule out malignancy ● Preoperative assessment for better evaluation of extent of tophi and their relation to adjacent anatomic structures ● Tophi have heterogeneous signal intensity, possibly hypointense on T2-weighted sequences ● Urate crystals have low signal intensity.
Soft tissues: Moderately increased signal intensity on T1-weighted images ● More markedly increased signal intensity on T2-weighted images ● Strongly enhancing.

Clinical Aspects

▶ **Typical presentation**
Clinical classification divided into four stages:
– Asymptomatic hyperuricemia (much more common than manifest gout).
– Acute gout.
– Intercritical stage (symptom-free interval between two attacks).
– Chronic gout with tophus formation and irreversible joint changes.

Acute gout: Sudden attack, often appearing at night, extremely painful monoarticular arthritis ● Redness ● Warmth ● Swelling ● Generalized signs of inflammation (fever, leukocytosis, increased ESR).

Chronic gout: Joint pain ● Gouty tophi ● Rarely occurs these days (in patients with inadequate treatment).

▶ **Treatment options**
  – Dietary: weight loss, low-purine diet, abstain from alcohol
  – Medication: NSAIDs and colchicine for acute gout ● Long-term treatment with uricostatic or uricosuric agents

▶ **Course and prognosis**
  Favorable prognosis with adequate prevention and treatment ● Untreated or insufficiently treated gout may lead to chronic joint and renal damage.

▶ **What does the clinician want to know?**
  Severity of articular lesions ● In some cases, confirmation of presumptive diagnosis.

Differential Diagnosis

Pseudogout	– Analysis of synovial fluid
	– No increase in uric acid concentration
	– Usually no erosive changes
Acute monoarticular arthritis/oligoarthritis	– Clinical presentation, no increase in uric acid concentration
	– Periostitis and bone apposition in seronegative spondylarthropathy
	– Erosive changes usually not well defined
Active osteoarthritis (first MTP joint)	– No erosive changes
	– Less pronounced soft-tissue swelling

Tips and Pitfalls

Misinterpreting lesions as signs of active osteoarthritis or acute monoarticular arthritis.

Selected References

Monu JU, Pope TL Jr. Gout: a clinical and radiologic review. Radiol Clin North Am 2004; 42(1): 169–184

Sheldon PJ, Forrester DM, Learch TJ. Imaging of intraarticular masses. Radiographics 2005; 25: 105–119

Uri DS, Dalinka MK Imaging of arthropathies. Crystal disease. Radiol Clin North Am 1996; 34(2): 359–374

Definition

Synonym: Bekhterev disease

▶ **Epidemiology**
Affects 0.2–0.3% of the population between ages 16 and 45 • Men affected seven times more often than women.

▶ **Etiology, pathophysiology, pathogenesis**
Seronegative spondylarthritis • Genetic predisposition • HLA-B27-positive.

Imaging Signs

▶ **Modality of choice**
Radiography • MRI in early stages.

▶ **Pathognomonic findings**
Syndesmophytes • Bamboo spine • Loss of anterior concavity of vertebral bodies • Sacroiliitis.

▶ **Radiographic/CT findings**
Vertebral column: Changes usually appear in the following order: Romanus lesions = "anterior spondylitis": osteitis of diskovertebral connection with erosions on anterior margins of vertebral bodies, less often also on posterior margins ("marginal spondylitis") • Square vertebrae (loss of anterior concavity of vertebral bodies due to inflammatory new bone formation along their anterior margins) • Syndesmophytes (ossifications in anulus fibrosus) • "Shiny corners": sclerotic healing of Romanus lesions • Andersson lesion: inflammatory/noninflammatory diskitis • Osteoporosis with ballooning of intervertebral disk • In late disease, development of "bamboo spine": ossifications in anulus fibrosus, ossification of longitudinal ligaments, supraspinous and interspinous ligaments, articular facets, joint capsule, and ligamenta flava • Disk calcifications • Complications: transverse fractures crossing the vertebral bodies or disk space and posterior elements (unstable, risk of paraplegia!), pseudarthrosis usually develops • Ankylosis of costovertebral joints with restricted breathing.
Sacroiliac joints: Inflammatory destructive changes • Indistinct joint contours • Erosions • More intense reactive sclerosis • Later ankylosis.
Calcaneus: Retrocalcaneal bursitis • Erosions at tendon attachment sites with subtle periostitis.
Peripheral arthritis: Incidence is 40% • Predilection for knee, hip, and shoulder joints • Radiographic signs resemble those of chronic polyarthritis.

▶ **MRI findings**
Imaging of early inflammatory changes involving the SI joint and spinal column • Bone marrow edema bordering SI joint (hyperintense on fat-saturated images, enhancing after contrast administration) • Diskitis (fluid signal in disk space) • Anterior spondylitis (inflammatory edema along anterior margin of vertebral body).

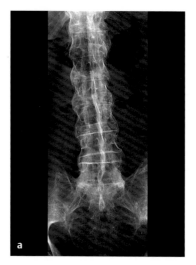 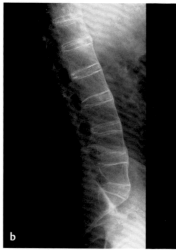

Fig. 2.13 a, b A 65-year-old man with long-standing ankylosing spondylitis. **a** AP and **b** lateral spinal radiographs. Typical "bamboo spine" appearance with syndesmophytes and ossification of the longitudinal ligaments as well as ankylosis of the sacroiliac joints.

Clinical Aspects

▶ **Typical presentation**
Chief symptoms are low back pain that occurs at night and morning stiffness (sacroiliitis) • Spinal stiffness • Iridocyclitis (30–50%) • Cardiac involvement • Pulmonary fibrosis • Colitis.

▶ **Treatment options**
Physical therapy • Nonsteroidal antirheumatic drugs • Glucocorticoids • Immunosuppressants.

▶ **Course and prognosis**
Chronic disease persisting for several decades • Highly variable level of severity • Spinal stiffening may be associated with significantly restricted motion and complications in later stages.

▶ **What does the clinician want to know?**
Evidence of sacroiliitis • Extent of spinal involvement • Fractures • Atlantoaxial instability.

Differential Diagnosis

Reiter syndrome	– Usually unilateral sacroiliitis, coarse parasyndesmophytes
Psoriasis	– Typical skin changes, peripheral joint involvement, coarse parasyndesmophytes

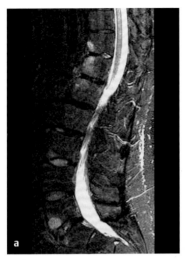
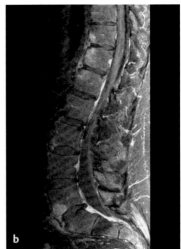

Fig. 2.14 a, b   A 39-year-old man with ankylosing spondylitis. MRI of the lumbar spine.
a STIR sequence showing multiple hyperintense inflammatory foci along the anterior margins of the vertebral bodies. Romanus lesions on L3 and L5. Anterior spondylitis of T11–L1.
b Postcontrast T1-weighted fat-saturated SE sequence showing marked enhancement of inflammatory lesions.

Rheumatoid arthritis	– Typical arthritic involvement of hands and feet
	– No syndesmophytes
	– In cervical spine involvement, stepladder deformity and erosion of spinous processes
DISH	– Large, bridging spondylophytes with preservation of disk space
	– No sacroiliitis

Tips and Pitfalls

Failing to recognize early disease ● Mistaking changes for "degeneration."

Selected References

Braun J, Sieper J. Ankylosing spondylitis [review]. Lancet 2007; 369(9570): 1379–1390
Levine DS, Forbat SM, Saifuddin A. MRI of the axial skeletal manifestations of ankylosing spondylitis [review]. Clin Radiol 2004; 59(5): 400–413
van der Heijde D, Landewe R, Hermann KG, et al; ASAS/OMERACT MRI in AS Working Group. Is there a preferred method for scoring activity of the spine by magnetic resonance imaging in ankylosing spondylitis? J Rheumatol 2007; 34(4): 871–873
Wendling D, Toussirot E, Streit G, Prati C. Imaging study scores for ankylosing spondylitis [review]. Joint Bone Spine 2006; 73(6): 655–660

Definition

▶ **Epidemiology**

1–3% of all pyogenic infections of the skeletal system ● First peak of disease incidence in early childhood ● Otherwise manifestation mainly in 5th and 6th decades ● No sex predilection ● Fatal in up to 5%.

▶ **Etiology, pathophysiology, pathogenesis**

Spondylitis is an inflammatory disease of the vertebrae ● "Spondylodiskitis" refers to infection of the disk space and adjacent vertebral body/bodies ● Usually caused by bacterial infection due to hematogenous spread, intervertebral disk surgery, or injection ● Rarely caused by invasion from surrounding tissues (e.g., retropharyngeal, presacral) abscess ● Pathogens: *Staphylococcus aureus*, *Streptococcus* sp., and *E. coli*, Gram-negative organisms in older patients with urinary tract infection, intestinal surgery, or intravenous drug use ● Predisposing factors include systemic disease such as diabetes mellitus as well as alcoholism and corticosteroid use ● Special variant: tuberculous spondylitis ● Predominantly affects lumbar and thoracic spine ● Cervical spine involvement less common in bacterial spondylitis.

Pathogenesis: Hematogenous spread to the bone marrow (especially near the well-vascularized end plates) ● Spread via intersegmental vessel branching to neighboring vertebral bodies ● Infection of avascular intervertebral disk by vessels perforating the end plates (through age 20) or (after age 20) vascularized periphery of the anulus fibrosus ● Usually monosegmental, rarely multisegmental (tuberculosis) ● Subligamentous spread or dissemination via Batson's plexus (communicating with pelvis) ● Spread into the paraspinal muscles ● Feared complications include invasion of paravertebral or epidural space (up to 20% lethality) and neurologic complications.

Imaging Signs

▶ **Modality of choice**

Radiographs ● MRI ● CT.

▶ **Radiographic findings**

In early disease, loss of intervertebral disk space height (NB: conventional radiographs are frequently false-negatives) ● Increasingly indistinct appearance of adjacent inferior and superior end plates ● As disease progresses, destruction of the end plates and anterior margin of the vertebral body ● During the course of healing, increasing sclerosis of the end plates and affected portions of the vertebral bodies.

▶ **CT findings**

Precise imaging of bony destruction ● In acute phase of disease, vertebral body fragmentation with moth-eaten appearance of vertebral end plates ● As disease progresses, reactive cancellous bone sclerosis ● Increased bone density ● Repair of erosions ● Paraspinal abscesses may occur ● CT-guided diskovertebral biopsy ● Abscess drainage.

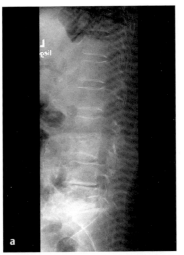

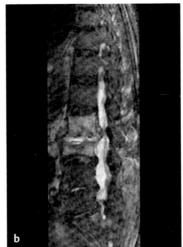

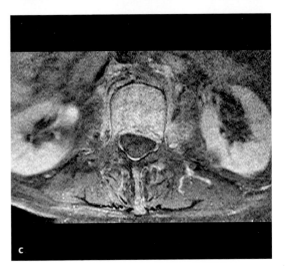

Fig. 2.15 a–c Spondylodiskitis affecting L2–L3 with abscess formation in the intervertebral disk space.

a Lateral radiograph showing loss of intervertebral disk space height between L2 and L3 and indistinct margins of the vertebral end plates.

b MRI, sagittal STIR sequence. Paravertebral spread of an abscess with suspected incipient involvement of the left psoas. Inflammatory changes in the epidural space.

c MRI, fat-saturated T1-weighted image after administration of contrast material.

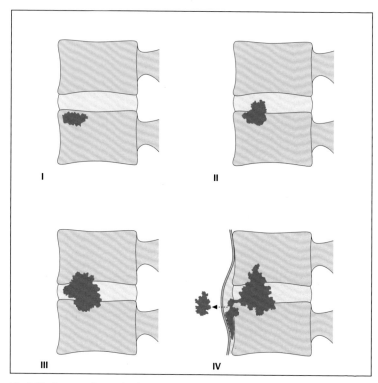

Fig. 2.16   Pattern of spread in hematogenous spondylodiskitis. The process starts with infection of well-vascularized portions of the vertebra near the vertebral end plates (I), leading to invasion of the intervertebral disk space (II). Abscess formation in the intervertebral disk space follows, with consequent loss of height (III). Spread continues into adjacent vertebral bodies, deep to the anterior/posterior longitudinal ligaments, and on into the paravertebral soft tissues (IV). Feared complications are epidural abscesses when infection continues to spread posteriorly.

▶ **MRI findings**
All sequences demonstrate high sensitivity (90–100%) • Signal isointense to fluid and rim enhancement imply disk abscess • Indistinct vertebral end plates • Changes typical of edema in surrounding vertebral bodies involving more than half of each affected vertebral body • Meningeal contrast enhancement • Epidural abscesses readily detected after administration of contrast material • Paravertebral spread is readily recognized.

Clinical Aspects

▶ **Typical presentation**
Localized back pain (increasing on percussion) • Radicular symptoms • Spinal cord symptoms • Fever • Elevated ESR, CRP, and white blood cell count.

▶ **Treatment options**
In uncomplicated spondylodiskitis, immobilization and parenteral antibiotics • Otherwise, surgical removal of diseased tissue • Isolate causative organism before initiating antibiotic treatment.

▶ **Course and prognosis**
Vertebral fusion in up to two-third of patients • Marked loss of height may occur • Kyphosis • Hump formation • Scoliosis.

▶ **What does the clinician want to know?**
Diagnosis • Stage • Location • Extent of disease • Paravertebral or epidural abscess formation.

Differential Diagnosis

Tumors	– Intervertebral disk spared – Often involve posterior vertebral elements
Osteochondrosis	– Vertebral end plates are more distinct – Edema usually involves less than half the vertebral body height – Lumbosacral junction typically affected

Tips and Pitfalls

Mistaking disease for one of the above-mentioned differential diagnoses.

Selected References

Longo M, Granata F, Ricciardi K, Gaeta M, Blandino A. Contrast-enhanced MR imaging with fat suppression in adult-onset septic spondylodiscitis. Eur Radiol 2003; 13(3): 626–637

Stabler A, Baur A, Kruger A, Weiss M, Helmberger T, Reiser M. Differential diagnosis of erosive osteochondrosis and bacterial spondylitis: magnetic resonance tomography (MRT) [in German]. Rofo 1998; 168(5): 421–428

Varma R, Lander P, Assaf A. Imaging of pyogenic infectious spondylodiskitis. Radiol Clin North Am 2001; 39(2): 203–213

Definition

Synonyms: reflex sympathetic dystrophy, algoneurodystrophy, complex regional pain syndrome (CRPS)

▶ **Epidemiology**

Post-traumatic in 90% after distal extremity fracture (incidence of 10–35% after Colles' fracture and 30% after tibial shaft fracture) ● Idiopathic in 10% ● Affects all age groups ● Peak incidence around age 50 ● Women affected twice as often as men.

▶ **Etiology, pathophysiology, pathogenesis**

Usually after (micro-)trauma or minor surgery on the extremities (e.g., carpal tunnel decompression, arthroscopy) ● Pathogenesis is poorly understood ● Disturbance of afferent and efferent nerves of the sympathetic nervous system as well as microcirculation ● Hyperactive sympathetic nervous system induces exaggerated regional inflammatory reaction.

Imaging Signs

▶ **Modality of choice**

Radiography, preferably with comparison view of contralateral side.

▶ **Radiographic/CT findings**

Only soft-tissue swelling in initial stages ● Bony changes visible at 4 weeks at the earliest and only detectable in 40% ● Patchy or band-like subchondral areas of decalcification ● Possible disappearance of subchondral bone end plate and cortical thinning due to bone resorption.

▶ **MRI findings**

No specific findings that assist diagnosis ● Suitable for ruling out other diseases ● In early stages, soft-tissue edema that enhances after contrast administration ● Bony structures usually remain unremarkable throughout disease course ● There may be focal or linear areas of patchy, slight edema, especially at subcortical sites ● These presumably represent secondary insufficiency fractures.

▶ **Nuclear medicine**

Scintigraphy with ^{99m}Tc-diphosphonate ● In disease stages 1 and 2, increased uptake in the soft-tissue phase (5–15 minutes after injection) and in the bone phase (after 3 hours) ● Increased tracer accumulation near the joints ● In stage 3 (atrophy), scintigram findings often normal.

▶ **Pathognomonic findings**

No pathognomonic features ● Usually patchy areas of decalcification in affected bones.

Clinical Aspects

▶ **Typical presentation**

Three stages in classic form of disease (though all are not always present):

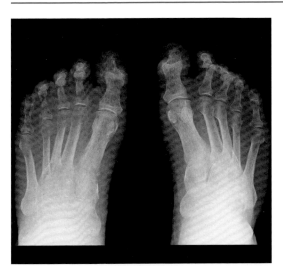

Fig. 2.17 An 87-year-old man after distal fibular fracture (Weber C fracture). Five weeks after removal of syndesmotic screws, dystrophic soft-tissue changes appeared. Radiograph of the right forefoot shows patchy and subchondral decalcifications indicative of CRPS.

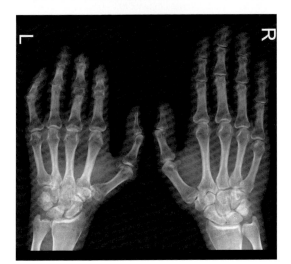

Fig. 2.18
A 50-year-old man 3 months after circular saw injury involving the second and third fingers of the left hand. Clinically typical CRPS with finger contractures. Radiographs of both hands. Comparison of sides reveals marked decalcification in the entire left hand and carpus, more pronounced around the joint.

- Stage I: Inflammation • Onset after days or weeks • Burning pain • Marked spontaneous pain and pain on weight-bearing • Swelling • Affected extremity is warmer or cooler than opposite side • Moist, warm, often shiny (bright red) skin • Hyperesthesia or hypesthesia • Hyperalgesia or hypalgesia • There may be increased hair growth and sweating.
- Stage II: Dystrophy • After weeks or months • Pain with movement and increasingly restricted range of motion • Mild pain at rest • Cool, dry skin that is pale or dark red to blue in color • Trophic changes • Contractures
- Stage III: Atrophy (irreversible) • Increasing dysfunction as a result of muscle atrophy • Fibrosis of capsules and ligaments • Atrophic, dry "waxy" skin • Anhydrosis • Contractures • Irreversible.

▶ **Treatment options**

Multidisciplinary treatment • Usually outpatient • Hospitalization may be necessary for pain therapy, physical therapy, ergotherapy, passive physical therapy, or psychotherapy • Bisphosphonates may be used.

▶ **Course and prognosis**

Variable course • On the whole, prognosis is unfavorable, although disease reversal is possible with rigorous, early treatment • Stage III disease is irreversible.

▶ **What does the clinician want to know?**

Signs of decalcification • Rule out differential diagnoses.

Differential Diagnosis
....

Disuse osteoporosis	– Homogeneous decalcification in affected skeletal area
	– No hyperperfusion on scintigraphy
	– No pain or soft-tissue swelling
Bone marrow edema syndrome	– Circumscribed area of edema in a bone
	– No clinically apparent soft-tissue injury
Osteomyelitis	– Radiographic appearance may be similar, but usually restricted to a single bone
	– On MRI, marked bone marrow changes

Tips and Pitfalls
....

May be difficult to distinguish from disuse osteoporosis.

Selected References

Berthelot JM. Current management of reflex sympathetic dystrophy syndrome (complex regional pain syndrome type I) [review]. Joint Bone Spine 2006; 73(5): 495–499

Intenzo CM, Kim SM, Capuzzi DM. The role of nuclear medicine in the evaluation of complex regional pain syndrome type I [review]. Clin Nucl Med 2005; 30(6): 400–407

Metz VM, Gilula LA. Imaging techniques for distal radius fractures and related injuries [review]. Orthop Clin North Am 1993; 24(2): 217–228

Definition

▶ **Epidemiology**
Important issue in social medicine ● Incidence as high as 80% in people aged 65 and over ● Most common sites of manifestation: hips, knees, hands ● Achilles tendon ● Oligoarticular or polyarticular disease.

▶ **Etiology, pathophysiology, pathogenesis**
Clinical syndrome comprising a heterogenous group of diseases all of which involve joint tissues ● Result of mechanical and biological events that disturb the normal balance of breakdown and synthesis of cartilage and subchondral bone.
 – Primary form: idiopathic.
 – Secondary form: post-traumatic ● Inflammatory ● Associated with congenital disorders ● Neuropathic.
 – Special variant: erosive osteoarthritis.
Multifactorial etiology ● Interactions between mechanisms (e.g., malalignment, neuromuscular malfunctions, ligamentous lesions (instability), trauma), and biological (enzymatic damage) factors ● Destruction of articular cartilage ● Subchondral bone remodeling ● Ultimately, destruction and restricted functioning of entire joint.
Cartilage changes: Damage to cartilage collagen fibers ● Reduced biosynthesis of chondrocytes ● Increasing fibrillation with loss of mechanical stability ● Synovitis and effusion induced by cartilage wear ● Further deterioration of cartilage leads to exposed areas of subchondral bone.
Periarticular changes: Subchondral marrow edema ● Microhemorrhage ● Reactive hyperemia ● Cell infiltration ● Formation of fibrovascular tissue ● Subchondral cysts ● Subchondral sclerosis ● Bone proliferation (osteophytes) caused by local activation of growth factors.
The menisci are also affected by joint degeneration.

Imaging Signs

▶ **Modality of choice**
Radiography ● CT ● MRI.

▶ **Radiographic findings**
Views in two planes ● Views of the knee should include weight-bearing images (AP standing view of knee) ● Joint space narrowing ● Osteophytes ● Subchondral sclerosis ● Subchondral cyst formation ● "Seagull" sign in erosive form involving the finger joints.
Classification: Kellgren–Lawrence (KL) grading system for hands, knees, and hips ● Scale ranges from 0 (no evidence of arthritis) to 4 (advanced-stage arthritis) ● Only limited correlation between clinical symptoms and KL grade.

▶ **CT findings**
Findings similar to radiography, but enable earlier detection without superimposition ● Useful for exclusion of intra-articular loose bodies (perhaps CT arthrography additionally) and chondrocalcinosis ● Imaging of complex bone structures (sacroiliac joints, acromioclavicular joints, small vertebral joints).

Kellgren–Lawrence (KL) osteoarthritis grading system

KL grade	Osteophytes	Joint space narrowing	Sclerosis
0	None	None	None
1	Doubtful	None	None
2	Mild	Possible	None
3	Moderate, several	Present	Possible
4	Large	Marked	Marked

▶ **MRI findings**

Detailed depiction of cartilage damage and meniscal changes • Subchondral changes (resembling bone marrow edema) in regions of altered mechanical stress • Correlation of changes with pain remains unclear • Reactive synovitis may be detected after contrast administration • Subchondral cysts and sclerosis • Smaller, necrotic areas in subchondral bone, usually in main weight-bearing zones.

Clinical Aspects

▶ **Typical presentation**

Pain • Limited range of motion • Morning stiffness • Symptoms worsen with weight-bearing • Symptoms reduce with cessation of weight-bearing • Crepitation.

Advanced stage: Swelling • Effusion • Malalignment • Subcutaneous soft-tissue nodules • Muscle tension • Ankylosis.

Erosive osteoarthritis: Swelling • Redness • Severe pain • Effusion.

These symptoms are summarized with radiological changes in the American College of Rheumatology (ACR) criteria for diagnosis of osteoarthritis.

▶ **Treatment options**

Treatment depends on stage, subjective complaints, age, and lifestyle • Conservative treatment in early stages, NSAIDs, intra-articular steroid injections • In advanced disease, management is surgical (e.g., osteotomy, microfracture, autologous chondrocyte or osteochondral transplantation, or joint replacement).

▶ **Course and prognosis**

Variable • Usually gradual development with increasingly limited function • Erosive osteoarthritis of DIP joints • In older patients with hip joint involvement, complete destruction may occur within a few weeks (Postel destructive coxarthrosis).

▶ **What does the clinician want to know?**

Extent of changes • Indication for surgery • Preoperative planning.

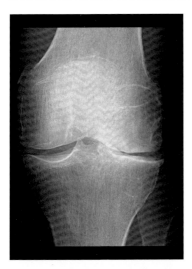

Fig. 3.1 Predominantly lateral femorotibial osteoarthritis. AP radiograph of the knee showing joint space narrowing, subchondral sclerosis, and central and peripheral osteophytes. Chondrocalcinosis evident as calcification at the attachment site of the medial collateral ligament after rupture several years previously.

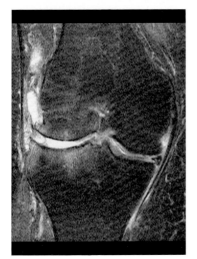

Fig. 3.2 Gonarthrosis. MRI (coronal, STIR) showing cartilage loss in the lateral compartment, joint effusion, meniscal degeneration, and subchondral bone edema, presumably as a reaction to inadequate biomechanics.

Differential Diagnosis

Rheumatoid disease	– Typical distribution pattern
	– Erosive changes
	– Clinical signs (CRP, duration of symptoms, morning stiffness)
	– Erosive/destructive changes also a prominent feature of secondary degenerative joint disease

Tips and Pitfalls

Grading of early osteoarthritis can be difficult in some cases.

Selected References

Buckland-Wright JC, Verbruggen G, Haraoui PB. Imaging. Radiological assessment of hand OA [review]. Osteoarthritis Cartilage 2000; 8(Suppl A): S55–56

Felson DT. An update on the pathogenesis and epidemiology of osteoarthritis. Radiol Clin North Am 2004; 42: 1–10

Haq I, Murphy E, Darce J. Osteoarthritis. Postgrad Med J 2003; 79: 377–383

Lang P, Noorbakhsh F, Yoshioka H. MR imaging of articular cartilage: current state and recent developments. Radiol Clin North Am 2005; 43(4): 629–639

Watt I. Arthrose – eine oder viele Erkrankungen? Radiologe 2000; 40: 1134–1140

Definition

▶ **Epidemiology**
Osteochondrosis is one of the most common sources of back pain ● Intervertebral disk degeneration is one of the main reasons for early retirement ● It is present in nearly 100% of people over age 70 ● Asymptomatic intervertebral disk degeneration is present in 35% of 20-year-olds (detectable on MRI).

▶ **Etiology, pathophysiology, pathogenesis**
Dehydration of the nucleus pulposus ● Fragmentation and tearing of anulus fibrosus ● Loss of intervertebral disk height ● Increased reactive sclerosis of vertebral end plates ● Possible complication: intervertebral disk prolapse ● Usually segmental hypomobility within a segment ● Possible segmental hypermobility as compensation in adjacent segment.

Imaging Signs

▶ **Modality of choice**
Radiography ● MRI.

▶ **Pathognomonic findings**
Decreased intervertebral disk height ● Sclerosis on adjacent vertebral end plates.

▶ **Radiographic findings**
Most usually affected are C5–C7 and L4–S1 ● Loss of intervertebral disk space height ● Increased sclerosis of adjacent superior and inferior vertebral end plates. Associated conditions include spondylarthritis, spondylosis, and spondylolisthesis.
Spondylarthritis: Arthritic changes affecting the facet joints ● Joint space narrowing ● Sclerosis of articular surfaces.
Spondylosis: Osteophytic lipping along vertebral end plates ● Osteophytes may cause neuroforaminal or spinal canal narrowing.
Spondylolisthesis: Vertebral body slip ● Vacuum phenomenon: completely degenerated intervertebral disk may allow leakage of nitrogen into the disk space, especially on extension ● Calcification of anterior and/or posterior longitudinal ligaments.

▶ **CT findings**
Concomitant disk herniation may be seen ● There may be spinal canal narrowing due to disk protrusion or prolapse ● Spondylarthritis ● Hypertrophy of ligamenta flava ● Calcifications in longitudinal ligaments.
Erosive osteochondrosis: Arises from microinstability of intervertebral disk ● Fibrovascular tissue grows into the hyaline cartilage end plates and intervertebral disk space ● This leads to irregular contouring of the inferior and superior end plates of the intervertebral disk.

▶ **MRI findings**
Intervertebral disk displays decreased signal intensity on T2-weighted images as a result of water loss ● Anular tear: punctate or linear signal increase in anulus fibrosus on T2-weighted SE images ● Modic classification of erosive osteochondrosis:

Fig. 3.3   A 58-year-old woman with marked osteochondrosis at L4–L5. Lateral radiograph of the lumbar spine showing loss of height of the disk space with a reactive, crescent-shaped area of bone sclerosis directly adjacent to the vertebral end plates. Vacuum phenomenon in the intervertebral disk space. Incidental finding of limbus vertebra at L5 (anterior disk herniation). Osteoarthritis of the facet joints L4–S1.

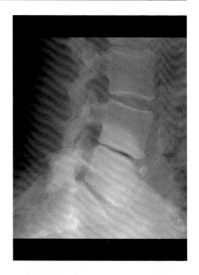

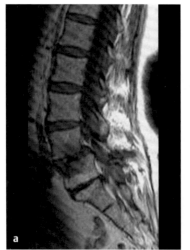
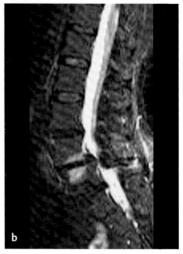

Fig. 3.4 a, b   A 60-year-old woman with erosive osteochondrosis (type I Modic changes) at L4–L5. MRI showing degenerative spondylolisthesis.

a   T1-weighted SE image showing hypointense band in the bone marrow along the vertebral end plates.

b   Fat-saturated STIR image. Hyperintense marrow signal consistent with edema.

– Type I Modic changes: vertebral end plate marrow edema • Band of hyperintense signal on T2-weighted or fat-saturated sequences • Hypointense signal on T1-weighted images.
– Type II Modic changes: fat deposits indicative of healing • Hyperintense signal on T1-weighted and T2-weighted images.
– Type III Modic changes: sclerosis • Hypointense signal on T1-weighted and T2-weighted images.

Clinical Aspects

▶ **Typical presentation**
Usually chronic, recurrent back pain without sensorimotor deficits • Erosive disease associated with severe symptoms (patients are unable get up when lying supine and have, for example, to roll onto one side to get out of bed).

▶ **Treatment options**
Passive physical therapy • Analgesics • Intervertebral fusion when microinstability is present, and pain cannot be managed conservatively.

▶ **Course and prognosis**
Erosive osteochondrosis usually heals within several months or years • Stiffness caused by spondylophytes (seen as fat deposits on MRI) • NB: Radiographic findings do not always correlate with clinical symptoms • Marked degenerative changes may be present even in patients who are virtually asymptomatic.

▶ **What does the clinician want to know?**
Extent of disk height loss • Active erosive osteochondrosis • Associated conditions: spondylosis, spondylarthritis, narrowing of the spinal canal or neuroforamina, disk protrusion/prolapse.

Differential Diagnosis

Spondylodiskitis	– Radiograph: vertebral end plates have indistinct borders and show sclerosis
	– MRI: fluid signal in disk space, epidural abscess, more marked edematous changes in adjacent vertebral bodies

Selected References

Haughton V. Imaging intervertebral disc degeneration [review]. J Bone Joint Surg Am 2006; 88(Suppl 2): 15–20
Jarvik JG, Deyo RA. Imaging of lumbar intervertebral disc degeneration and aging, excluding disc herniations [review]. Radiol Clin North Am 2000; 38(6): 1255–1266
Niosi CA, Oxland TR. Degenerative mechanics of the lumbar spine. Spine 2004; 4: 202–208
Paarjanen H, Erkintalo M, Kuusela T, Dahlstrom S, Kormano M. Magnetic resonance study of disc degeneration in young low-back pain patients. Spine 1989; 14: 982–985
Pfirrman CWA, Metzdorf A, Zanetti M, Hodler J, Boos N. Magnetic resonance classification of lumbar intervertebral disc degeneration. Spine 2001; 26(17): 1873–1878

Definition

▶ **Epidemiology**
Incidence is unknown • Disk herniation is detectable in up to one-third of asymptomatic adults • In Germany, the rate of intervertebral disk surgery is 87 per 100 000 inhabitants.

▶ **Etiology, pathophysiology, pathogenesis**
Anular tear related to aging process • Excessive pressure in nucleus pulposus leads to disk protrusion (outer portions of the anulus fibrosus as well as posterior longitudinal ligament remain intact) • Later, disk herniation with displacement of portions of the nucleus pulposus and/or anulus into the epidural space.
– Intervertebral disk protrusion: focal or circular.
– Focal disk protrusion: focal protrusion of outer disk contour due to herniation of nucleus pulposus material into the anulus fibrosus (outer portions of the anulus fibrosus remain intact) • Precursor to disk herniation.
– Concentric disk protrusion: broad-based protrusion of the anulus fibrosus peripherally • Usually circular or semicircular • Caused by dehydration and thus loss of pressure in nucleus pulposus • Not a precursor to disk herniation.
– Disk herniation/prolapse/extrusion: herniation of disk tissue beyond the periphery of the anulus fibrosus into the spinal canal.

Imaging Signs

▶ **Modality of choice**
MRI • Alternatively, CT/CT myelography.

▶ **Pathognomonic findings**
Herniation of nucleus pulposus tissue into the spinal canal • Biconvex protrusion of anulus fibrosus posteriorly (axial images) • Disk tissue above and/or below the level of the vertebral end plates.

▶ **Radiographic findings**
Herniation cannot be visualized directly • Unreactive decreased intervertebral space height and scoliosis due to pain may be indirect signs.

▶ **CT findings**
CT useful if MRI is not available or cannot be performed • CT will show bony canal narrowing caused by spondylophytes • Herniated disk visible as an extradural mass in the anterior portion of the spinal canal which is isodense to soft tissue (70 HU) and has contact with the intervertebral disk in the intervertebral space • Sagittal reconstructions can assist in determining the affected segment.

▶ **MRI findings**
Modality of choice: sagittal T1-weighted and T2-weighted TSE sequences, axial (parallel to inferior and superior vertebral end plates of adjacent vertebral bodies) and coronal T2-weighted SE sequences • Coronal sequences allow precise assessment of level (last costovertebral joint).
Anular tear: T2-weighted images show focal or linear signal increase in the hypointense anulus fibrosus • There is usually contrast enhancement of fibrovascular, healing tissue which projects into the fissure.

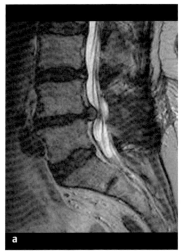

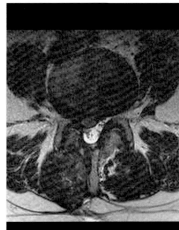

Fig. 3.5 a–c   A 59-year-old woman 2 months after intervertebral disk surgery at L4–L5. MRI.

a   Sagittal T2-weighted TSE. Readily identifiable recurrent disk prolapse. Additional anular tear (hyperintense focal lesion in the dorsal portion of the anulus fibrosus) at the level of L3–L4.

b   Axial T2-weighted TSE. Herniated disk on the right mediolateral side.

c   After administration of contrast material, peripheral enhancement of the prolapsed disk. Edematous, enhancing posterior soft tissues (recent scar tissue).

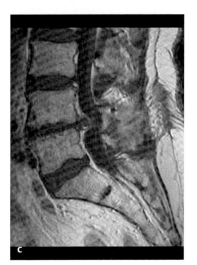

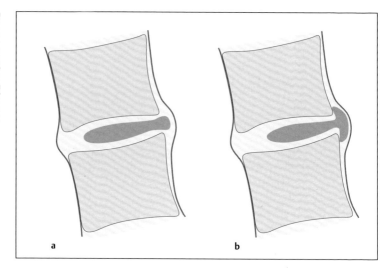

Fig. 3.6 a, b Intervertebral disk protrusion (**a**) and extrusion (**b**). In extrusion (as against protrusion), disk tissue extends cranially or caudally past the level of the vertebral end plates.

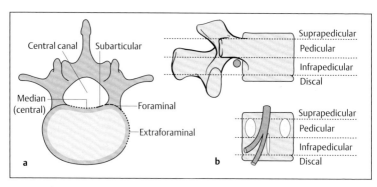

Fig. 3.7 a, b Horizontal and craniocaudal positional relationships of a herniated disk.

Disk protrusion: Biconcave posterior protrusion of the anulus fibrosus (axial images) • Disk tissue lies above and/or below the level of the vertebral end plates (sagittal views) • Hyperintense nucleus pulposus material herniates posteriorly beyond the margin of the anular fibers into the spinal canal • Disk material itself is nonenhancing • In the periphery of the hernia, contrast enhancement is possible due to secondary vascularization of the intervertebral disk or expanded epidural venous plexus • Nucleus pulposus tissue may lie along the posterior aspect of the anulus, resembling a protrusion (peripheral hyperintense zone on T1-weighted and T2-weighted images, adjacent to hypointense anular fibers).

Position of the disk material must be described precisely • On axial images: medial, mediolateral, lateral; in lateral recess, intraforaminal, lateral; extraforaminal • Extent of tear in craniocaudal plane: at disk level, infrapedicular, pedicular, suprapedicular • Subligamentous or transligamentous (penetration of posterior longitudinal ligament).

Sequestered disk: Cranially or caudally displaced herniated disk tissue that may or may not be connected to the disk of origin • Disk material generally located behind the vertebral body, but may extend to the intervertebral foramen.

Intravertebral hernia: Schmorl nodule • Herniation of disk material into the vertebral body through a defect in the hyaline cartilage end plate.

▶ **Myelographic findings**
Useful supplementary study only in exceptional situations, e.g., discrepancy between clinical symptoms and noncontrast CT and/or MRI studies • Nonenhancing structure in the epidural space at the level of the intervertebral disk space • Nerve roots possibly shortened and/or displaced by the mass.

Clinical Aspects

▶ **Typical presentation**
Depends on affected spinal level, position, and size of herniation • Lumbago and radicular pain • Sensory disturbances and pareses also possible in the area supplied by affected nerve roots.

▶ **Treatment options**
Conservative treatment: Only in patients without recent paresis or symptoms of cauda equina syndrome • Combination of pain therapy (NSAIDs, steroids, opioids) and passive physical therapy (physical therapy, hot compresses, massage).

Minimally invasive techniques: Only in patients without motor deficits or bladder/rectal dysfunction • Epidural injections • Catheter.

Surgical management: Indicated when pain is not manageable with conservative treatment or when pareses are present • Absolute indications: recent motor dysfunction and cauda equina syndrome (urinary/rectal dysfunction, sexual dysfunction, "saddle" anesthesia).

▶ **Course and prognosis**
Spontaneous resolution of disk herniation is possible (35% of cases) • "Failed back surgery syndrome": recurrence of radicular symptoms after surgery, caused

by recurrent herniation, scar tissue, spondylodiskitis, or erosive osteochondrosis with mechanical microinstability.

▶ **What does the clinician want to know?**

Height • Position • Nerve root compression • Narrowing of a neuroforamen • Sequestration • Junction anomalies • Correlation between radiological findings and neurological symptoms • Rule out differential diagnoses: bony spinal canal stenosis, tumor, abscess.

Differential Diagnosis

Epidural abscess	– Usually extending over several levels
	– Peripherally enhancing after contrast administration
	– Usually also symptoms of spondylodiskitis
Spondylophyte	– Bony outgrowth along vertebral margin
	– Mainly detectable on CT

Tips and Pitfalls

– Sequestrum missed in the neuroforamen. The entire neuroforamen should be shown on sagittal MRI sections.
– Symptoms not correlated with the level of the radiological findings. This leads to "failed back surgery syndrome" when the cause of pain (e.g., erosive osteochondrosis or active spondylarthritis) is not eliminated.
– Incorrect identification of level of spinal involvement (especially with rib anomalies at T12 or junction anomalies), hence importance of coronal images.

Selected References

Babar S, Saifuddin A. MRI of the post-discectomy lumbar spine [review]. Clin Radiol 2002; 57(11): 969–981

Fardon DF, Milette PC; Combined Task Forces of the North American Spine Society, American Society of Spine Radiology, and American Society of Neuroradiology. Nomenclature and classification of lumbar disc pathology. Recommendations of the Combined Task Forces of the North American Spine Society, American Society of Spine Radiology, and American Society of Neuroradiology. Spine 2001; 26(5): E93–E113

McCall IW. Lumbar herniated discs [review]. Radiol Clin North Am 2000; 38(6): 1293–1309

Milette PC. Classification, diagnostic imaging, and imaging characterization of a lumbar herniated disc [review]. Radiol Clin North Am 2000; 38(6): 1267–1292

Milette PC. The proper terminology for reporting lumbar intervertebral disorders. AJNR Am J Neuroradiol 1997; 18(10): 1859–1866

Zhou Y, Abdi S. Diagnosis and minimally invasive treatment of lumbar discogenic pain—a review of the literature. Clin J Pain 2006; 22(5): 468–481

Definition

▶ **Epidemiology**
Incidence of 5 in 100 000 • No sex predilection.

▶ **Etiology, pathophysiology, pathogenesis**
Spinal canal width cannot accommodate volume of nerve roots/spinal cord •
Rarely, congenital narrowing, e.g., increased incidence in patients with achondroplasia • Usually degenerative (secondary) • Predominantly affects lumbar spine • Narrowing of spinal canal due to arthritic changes involving facet joints, spondylophytes, ligamenta flava hypertrophy, disk protrusion/prolapse, spondylolisthesis, epidural lipomatosis, calcified posterior longitudinal ligament (especially in cervical regions) • Monosegmental or multisegmental involvement.

Imaging Signs

▶ **Modality of choice**
CT myelography • MRI.

▶ **Pathognomonic findings**
Subarachnoid space disappears on MRI and CT myelography • Narrowing of spinal canal due to disk tissue, spondylarthritis, and hypertrophy of the ligamenta flava.

▶ **Radiographic findings**
Lateral views reveal narrowed sagittal diameter of the spinal canal • Cervical stenosis likely when sagittal diameter < 1.5 cm (measured from posterior margin of vertebral body to anterior base of spinous process) and transverse diameter < 2.0 cm (interpedicular distance) • Signs include osteochondrosis, posterior spondylophytes, spondylarthritis.

▶ **Myelographic findings**
Introduction of nonionic, water-soluble contrast material into the subarachnoid space • Puncture is usually at the level of L3–L4 and must be below the conus region (T12–L1) • Lateral, AP, and oblique (nerve root amputation) views as well as lateral standing views and dynamic flexion–extension views (effect of weight-bearing on the spinal canal width; demonstration of instability) • Spinal narrowing usually increases on posterior flexion at the level of the intervertebral disk spaces • This functional assessment is important for surgical planning.

▶ **Postmyelography CT findings**
CT scan is performed after myelography • Excellent depiction of narrowing due to contrast-containing dural sac • Absolute lumbar spinal stenosis is present when subarachnoid space is "lost" • A distinction is made between:
– Central spinal stenosis.
– Stenosis of the lateral recess and foramina.
– Intervertebral stenosis.

▶ **MRI findings**
Optimal imaging of the spinal canal (subarachnoid space) and diskoligamentous structures • In absolute stenosis, subarachnoid space is "lost" • Cauda equina fibers proximal to the stenosis are elongated and wavy • Compression-induced radiculitis may be present: thickened, edematous nerve roots.

Fig. 3.8   A 69-year-old woman with long-standing pain in the lumbar region and typical spinal claudication. Postmyelography CT scan (sagittal reconstruction). High-grade spinal stenosis at L4–L5 and L5–S1 caused by intervertebral disk protrusion, facet joint arthritis, and hypertrophy of the ligamenta flava.

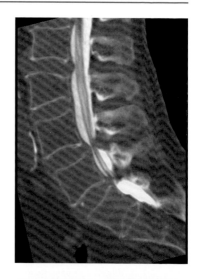

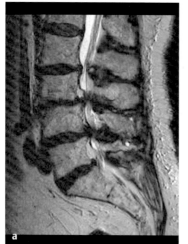
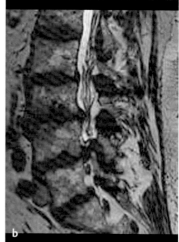

Fig. 3.9 a, b   An 80-year-old man with absolute spinal canal stenosis at L3–L4 and L4–L5.
a Sagittal T2-weighted TSE image. Spinal canal stenosis due to concentric disk protrusion, spondylarthritis, and hypertrophy of the ligamenta flava.
b Sagittal constructive interference in steady state (CISS) sequence with 1 mm slice thickness. The cauda equina fibers located cranial to the stenosis have a typical elongated and wavy appearance.

Clinical Aspects

▶ **Typical presentation**
Spinal claudication: pain radiating from lumbar region or buttocks into the thighs • Usually feeling of weakness or heaviness, especially when walking up an incline (hyperlordosis) • Presence of nerve root compression may cause sensory disturbances and pareses • Symptoms alleviated with spinal flexion • Bicycle riding often possible (in contrast to differential diagnosis of intermittent claudication).

▶ **Treatment options**
Acute: Kyphotic positioning (using foam blocks) • Antiphlogistic drugs.
Chronic: Stabilizing, antilordotic physical therapy • For therapy-resistant disease, epidural steroid administration may be attempted • Where height of anterior disk elements and soft-tissue components is preserved, minimally invasive treatment with interspinous implants may be tried • Otherwise, depending on severity of stenosis and instability, treat with decompression (microscopically assisted fenestration with undercutting or laminectomy, with or without spondylodesis).

▶ **Course and prognosis**
Natural course: condition worsens in 15% after 4 years • Improvement in 15% • In 70% symptoms remain stable • Controversy surrounding various surgical measures.

▶ **What does the clinician want to know?**
Localization of narrowing • Absolute or relative stenosis • Monosegmental or multisegmental • Central, lateral recess, or foraminal stenosis • Dynamic myelography.

Differential Diagnosis

Intervertebral disk prolapse – Anterior narrowing of dural sac caused by disk tissue

Tips and Pitfalls

Underestimating the degree of stenosis with failure to obtain functional assessment projections (with patient standing) after myelography (which should include flexion–extension views) • Mistaking spinal stenosis for intermittent claudication in peripheral vascular occlusive disease.

Selected References

de Graaf I, Prak A, Bierma-Zeinstra S, Thomas S, Peul W, Koes B. Diagnosis of lumbar spinal stenosis: a systematic review of the accuracy of diagnostic tests [review]. Spine 2006; 31(10): 1168–1176

Jinkins JR. MR evaluation of stenosis involving the neural foramina, lateral recesses, and central canal of the lumbosacral spine [review]. Magn Reson Imaging Clin N Am 1999; 7(3):493–511, viii

Saifuddin A. The imaging of lumbar spinal stenosis [review]. Clin Radiol 2000; 55(8): 581–594

Definition

▶ **Epidemiology**

Incidence is 3–6% ● Low incidence among black women (1.1%) ● Most commonly found in white men (6.4%) ● In 85–95% disease affects L5, followed by L4 (5–15%) and L3 ● Unilateral or bilateral involvement.

▶ **Etiology, pathophysiology, pathogenesis**

Cleft in pars interarticularis of vertebral arch ● Suggested causes include a combination of hereditary weakness and stress/fatigue fracture (hyperextension movements, e.g., in artistic gymnastics) ● Usually manifests during childhood ● Associated with spina bifida ● Development of defects often leads to spondylolisthesis (slippage of a vertebral body).

Imaging Signs

▶ **Modality of choice**

Radiographs of lumbar spine in two planes, supplementary oblique views at 45° angle ● CT if defect not visible radiographically.

▶ **Pathognomonic findings**

Defect in the pars articularis with listhesis in this segment ● In acute spondylolysis, edema on MRI.

▶ **Radiographic/CT findings**

Defect in the pars articularis, sometimes with adjacent reactive sclerosis ● "Scotty dog" with collar ● Radiography may yield false-negatives.

Secondary signs: Sclerosis along contralateral pedicle ● Spondylolisthesis: displacement of a vertebral body relative to that immediately below it ● Either anterolisthesis (forward slippage) or retrolisthesis (backward slippage) ● Classification of extent of spondylolisthesis based on Meyerding's system (grades 1–4: one-quarter to four-quarters of the sagittal diameter of the vertebral body).

▶ **CT findings**

More sensitive than conventional radiography for detection of lytic areas ● Often adjacent reactive sclerosis or callus formation.

▶ **MRI findings**

Modality of choice in the acute phase ● In the acute stage, pedicles and pars interarticularis demonstrate slightly hyperintense signal on fat-saturated images (bone marrow edema) ● Actual fracture: disruption in pars interarticularis which appears as a hypointense band on T1-weighted and T2-weighted images ● In older fractures pars interarticularis demonstrates reactive sclerosis (hypointense on T1-weighted and T2-weighted images).

▶ **Nuclear medicine**

Differentiates between recent and older spondylolysis ● Increased uptake in recent or imminent fatigue fracture ● Older fractures rarely demonstrate tracer accumulation ● High sensitivity ● Low specificity.

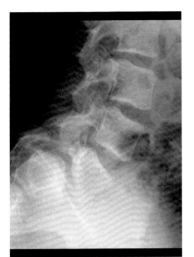

Fig. 3.10   Spondylolysis of pars interarticularis in a 14-year-old boy with low back pain. Lateral radiograph of the lumbar spine showing marked spondylolisthesis at L5–S1 (Meyerding grade 3).

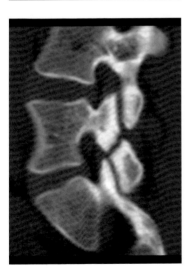

Fig. 3.11   A 26-year-old man with a 2-year history of left lumbar pain radiating into the buttocks and no radicular symptoms. Sagittal reconstruction of CT images. Spondylolysis of pars interarticularis at L5–S1. No evidence of spondylolisthesis.

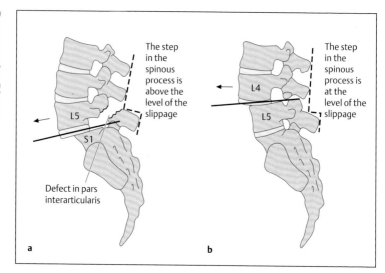

Fig. 3.12 a, b   Spondylolysis with **a** spondylolisthesis and **b** pseudospondylolisthesis in vertebral degeneration.

Clinical Aspects

▶ **Typical presentation**
   Low back pain that intensifies on extension • Patients may be asymptomatic • Occasionally nerve root irritation.

▶ **Treatment options**
   Choice of therapy depends on patient age, disease severity, and localization.
   Conservative treatment: Physical therapy to strengthen muscles that stabilize the trunk, especially abdominal muscles (antilordotic exercises) • Passive physical therapy • Short-term bracing (corset).
   Surgical management: Interbody fusion • Indications: pain that cannot be managed conservatively, postural problems, progressive slippage or severe forward translation, neurologic deficit.

▶ **Course and prognosis**
   Prognosis is usually good • Defect becomes bridged with fibrocartilaginous tissue • Complications include spinal stenosis and pseudarthrosis with instability.

▶ **What does the clinician want to know?**
   Presence of defects • Extent of slippage • Spinal canal narrowing • Associated degenerative changes.

Differential Diagnosis

Degenerative spondylolisthesis	– Vertebral slippage without defect in pars interarticularis
	– Occurs in osteochondrosis and facet joint degeneration

Tips and Pitfalls

On axial CT images, a fissure may be mistaken for the facet joint directly below it; hence always obtain sagittal reconstructions.

Selected References

Campbell RSD, Grainger AJ, Hide IG, Papastefanou S, Greenough CG. Juvenile spondylolysis: a comparative analysis of CT, SPECT and MRI. Skeletal Radiol 2005; 34(2): 63–73

Ulmer JL, Mathews VP, Elster AD, Mark LP, Daniels DL, Mueller W. MR Imaging of lumbar spondylolysis: the importance of ancillary observations. AJR Am J Roentgenol 1997; 169(1): 233–239

Definition

▶ **Epidemiology**
Hip and knee prostheses have a lifetime of up to 20 years ● Up to 1% show loosening after 10 years.

▶ **Etiology, pathophysiology, pathogenesis**
Infection (septic loosening, early complication, i.e., within first 3 months after surgery) ● Mechanical factors (late complications).

Imaging Signs

▶ **Modality of choice**
Radiographs in two planes.

▶ **Radiographic findings**
Signs of loosening in cementless implants:
- Radiolucent line around more than one-third of the prosthesis circumference at the bone/prosthesis boundary (2 mm width or more is significant) that is progressively increasing in size ● The larger the radiolucent zone, the greater the index of suspicion.
- Change in position of prosthesis material ● Any change greater than 5 mm or 5° is considered a sign of loosening.

Signs of loosening in cemented implants:
- Radiolucent line between the bone and cement that is increasing with time.
- Gap between cement and prosthesis suggesting lack of contact and thus a weak bond between prosthesis and cement.
- Change in position of prosthesis material relative to cement.
- Breaks along cement mantle and changes in position of cement in medullary cavity.

▶ **Arthrography findings**
Leakage of contrast material between the bone/cement and the prosthesis after intra-articular injection of contrast material is evidence of loosening ● If no leakage is evident, rule out occult implant loosening with delayed-phase image after 30 minutes of weight-bearing ● Prior to administering contrast agent, obtain a sample of joint fluid for microbiological analysis.

▶ **Nuclear medicine**
Tracer accumulation is a sign of loosening ● Aseptic loosening due to mechanical causes tends to have focal tracer uptake ● Diffuse uptake around prosthesis circumference implies septic loosening ● Interpretation is often difficult given that, even in clinically asymptomatic patients, accumulation may be evident more than 1 year after surgery.

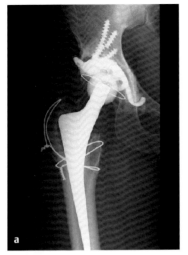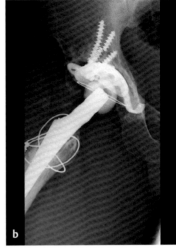

Fig. 3.13 a, b Loosening of acetabular cup after total hip replacement. **a** AP and **b** axial radiographs. Broken anchoring screws indicate instability and loosening of the cup. Tension band wiring around the greater trochanter after fracture during surgery. Mild periarticular ossification.

Clinical Aspects

▸ **Typical presentation**
Pain ● Restricted range of motion ● If infection present, redness, swelling, effusion.
▸ **Treatment options**
Revision surgery.
▸ **Course and prognosis**
Depends on age, mechanical stresses, bone, type of prosthesis.
▸ **What does the clinician want to know?**
Signs of loosening.

Differential Diagnosis

Cement retraction	– Radiolucent zone usually less than 2 mm wide that remains constant over time

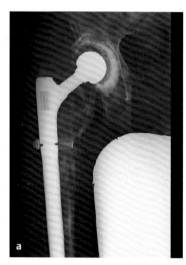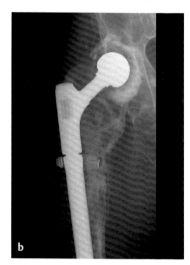

Fig. 3.14 a, b Acetabular revision surgery after total hip replacement.
a AP radiograph showing radiolucent line between cement and acetabulum. Cerclage wiring of femoral shaft due to periprosthetic fracture.
b AP radiograph 1 year later. Cerclage wiring has migrated. Prosthesis shaft has migrated laterally out of the femur. In addition, the now more sharply tilted acetabulum indicates renewed acetabular loosening.

Tips and Pitfalls

Initial loosening is easily missed, especially in patients with marked osteopenia, and may be mistaken for cement retraction.

Selected References

DeLee JG, Charnley J. Radiological demarcation of cemented sockets in total hip replacement. Clin Orthop 1976; (121): 20–32

Gruen TA, McNeice GM, Amstutz HC. "Modes of failure" of cemented stem-type femoral components. A radiographic analysis of loosening. Clin Orthop 1979; (141): 17–27

Definition (DISH, Forestier Disease)

▶ **Epidemiology**
Incidence is 3–15% • Men slightly more often affected than women • Usually manifests after age 50.

▶ **Etiology, pathophysiology, pathogenesis**
Etiology unknown • More common among patients who are obese or who have diabetes mellitus or hyperuricemia.

Imaging Signs

▶ **Modality of choice**
Radiography.

▶ **Pathognomonic findings**
"Dripping candle wax" appearance produced by osteophytic growths that bridge several vertebral segments while intervertebral disk space width seems relatively normal.

▶ **Radiographic findings**
"Dripping candle wax" appearance formed by osteophytes on the anterior aspects of the vertebral bodies bridging four or more vertebral bodies • Relatively unremarkable disk spaces, intervertebral joints, and SI joints • Ossification of fibrous tissue, i.e., new bone formation at sites of fibro-osseous transition.

▶ **CT findings**
As radiographic findings • May involve calcification of posterior longitudinal ligament leading to spinal canal narrowing.

▶ **MRI findings**
MRI indicated for diagnosis of myelopathy (increased spinal cord signal on T2-weighted images).

Clinical Aspects

▶ **Typical presentation**
Sometimes an incidental finding in asymptomatic patients • Sometimes associated with limited range of motion, especially in cervical spine or lower thoracic spine involvement.

▶ **Treatment options**
No satisfactory treatment to date • Physical therapy and analgesics • Surgical removal of osteophytes as a last resort in patients with complications.

▶ **Course and prognosis**
Chronic, progressive disease associated with increasingly limited range of motion • Fracture of ossifications • Extensive osteophytes on cervical spine may cause difficulty in swallowing • Intubation anesthesia is problematic • Calcification of posterior longitudinal ligament can lead to narrowing of spinal canal and potential myelopathy.

Fig. 3.15 A 67-year-old man with DISH at the thoracolumbar junction. Radiograph showing "dripping candle wax" appearance of spondylophytes bridging the vertebrae. Intervertebral disk space width remains relatively normal.

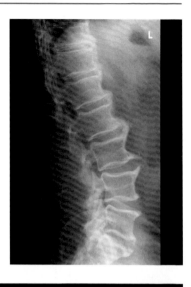

Fig. 3.16 DISH. Pelvic radiograph showing brush-like bony proliferations at the tendon attachments on the iliac crest consistent with ossification of fibrous tissue.

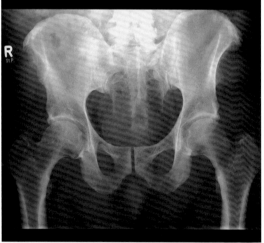

▶ **What does the clinician want to know?**
Distinguish from spondylosis and ankylosing spondylitis • Peripheral involvement • Progression of ossification over time • Complications.

Differential Diagnosis

Spondylosis	– Beak-like osteophytic structures on the vertebral bodies in degenerative changes of intervertebral disk space with disk height loss
	– Usually accompanied by spondylarthritis
Ankylosing spondylitis	– Syndesmophytes (tiny calcifications in anulus fibrosus)
	– Arthritis of SI joint

Tips and Pitfalls

Mistaking disease for spondylosis deformans.

Selected References

Cammisa M, De Serio A, Guglielmi G. Diffuse idiopathic skeletal hyperostosis [review]. Eur J Radiol 1998; 27(Suppl 1): S7–11

Hoffman LE, Taylor JA, Price D, Gertz G. Diffuse idiopathic skeletal hyperostosis (DISH): a review of radiographic features and report of four cases. J Manipulative Physiol Ther 1995; 18(8): 547–553

Mader R. Diffuse idiopathic skeletal hyperostosis: a distinct clinical entity [review]. Isr Med Assoc J 2003; 5(7): 506–508

Sarzi-Puttini P, Atzeni F. New developments in our understanding of DISH (diffuse idiopathic skeletal hyperostosis) [review]. Curr Opin Rheumatol 2004; 16(3): 287–292

Definition

▶ **Epidemiology**

Most common cause is diabetic foot syndrome ● Prevalence of Charcot foot without ulceration in diabetics is 0.2% (about 16 000 patients in Germany) ● Frequently encountered in specialized foot clinics.

▶ **Etiology, pathophysiology, pathogenesis**

Causes include diabetes mellitus, syphilis, leprosy, syringomyelia, and spina bifida with meningomyelocele ● Acute or chronic articular destruction by means of disrupted neurovascular supply of bone and soft tissues ● Changes resemble those in osteoarthritis, but in its most severe form ● Fragmentation of bone and cartilage ● Fragments are ground down to joint debris ● Resulting synovitis and effusion ● (Sub-)luxation often occurs.

Imaging Signs

▶ **Modality of choice**

Radiography ● MRI.

▶ **Radiographic findings**

Marked destruction and joint disintegration in patients with related underlying disease, predominantly diabetes.

▶ **Radiographic findings**

In diabetic patients, predilection for the foot ● In syringomyelia, preference for upper extremity (shoulder joint).

Early (active) stage: Demineralization or osteolysis near the joint ● Joint space narrowing ● Articular surface collapse ● Insufficiency fractures.

Late (reparative) chronic stage: Sclerosis of affected bones ● Osteophytes ● Subluxation ● Bone debris within the joint ● Synostosis/ankylosis.

Classification of diabetic foot after Eichenholtz:

– Stage I: Radiographic findings negative or show localized osteoporosis.
– Stage II: Coalescence of small bone fragments ● Absorption of fine bone debris.
– Stage III: Consolidation and remodeling of fracture fragments.

▶ **MRI findings**

Detection of soft-tissue and bone marrow edema (hypointense on T1-weighted images, hyperintense on fat-saturated sequences) ● Synovial enhancement after administration of contrast agent (synovitis) ● Joint effusion.

▶ **Nuclear medicine**

Tracer accumulation (Tc diphosphate complexes), especially during the delayed phase.

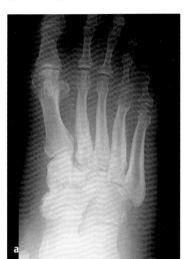

Fig. 3.17 a, b Neuropathic osteoarthropathy of the foot in a 69-year-old man with long-standing diabetes mellitus.
a Radiograph of the foot showing sites of bony destruction on the base of the second metatarsal. Osteosclerotic changes affecting the scaphoid toward the medial cuneiform and on the intermediate cuneiform toward the second metatarsal.
b T1-weighted MRI after contrast administration showing soft-tissue edema and edematous tarsal bones as well as cystic changes and synovitis.

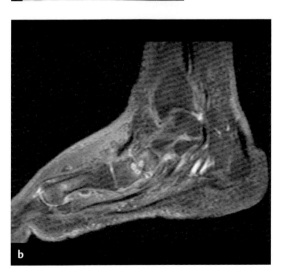

Clinical Aspects

▶ **Typical presentation**
Worsening joint pain ● Sometimes swelling ● Hyposensitivity of patients usually results in considerable discrepancy between striking radiological findings and low level of subjective symptoms.

▶ **Treatment options**
Orthotic devices ● Avoid pressure points ● Skin care.

▶ **Course and prognosis**
Usually progressive.

▶ **What does the clinician want to know?**
Affected joints ● Rule out osteomyelitis.

Differential Diagnosis

Osteomyelitis	– May be difficult to distinguish given similar patient profiles and clinical presentation
	– Radiographs: rapid disintegration of bone, gas foci
	– Scintigraphy: hyperperfusion in early phase of two-phase bone scan
	– MRI: formations typical of abscesses, sinus tracts leading to superficial skin ulcers. Limited to the affected foot compartment. Otherwise, signal alterations very similar to those in neurogenic osteoarthropathy with edematous soft tissues and bones
Osteoarthritis	– Focally narrowed joint space
	– Subchondral sclerosis
	– Osteophytes, but usually no joint destruction or (sub-)luxation
	– No bone debris

Tips and Pitfalls

Mistaking disease for osteomyelitis or osteoarthritis.

Selected References

Eichenholtz SN. Charcot joints. Springfield, Ill.: Charles C. Thomas, 1966

Gold RH, Tong DJF, Crim JR, Seeger LL. Imaging the diabetic foot. Skeletal Radiol 1995; 24(8): 563–572

Sinha S, Munichoodappa C, Kozak GP. Neuro-arthropathy (Charcot joints) in diabetes mellitus: a clinical study of 101 cases. Medicine 1972; 51(3): 191–210

Definition

▶ **Epidemiology**
Affects one in three women and one in eight men worldwide ● Prevalence among women three times high as among men.

▶ **Etiology, pathophysiology, pathogenesis**
Systemic bone disease ● Low bone mass ● Abnormal osseous microarchitecture ● Result is increased fracture risk.
– Type 1: Postmenopausal osteoporosis ● Result of estrogen and testosterone deficiency.
– Type 2: Senile osteoporosis (> 70 years of age).
– Type 3: Secondary osteoporosis ● Caused by medications (e.g., glucocorticoids, phenytoin) or diseases that lead to bone loss (e.g., Cushing disease, hyperparathyroidism, hyperthyroidism, hypogonadism, intestinal malabsorption, multiple myeloma).

Imaging Signs

▶ **Modality of choice**
Dual-energy X-ray absorptiometry (DXA) ● Alternatively, quantitative CT (QCT).

▶ **Pathognomonic findings**
Radiographs show increased radiolucency ● Codfish vertebrae or wedged vertebrae ● Insufficiency fractures ● DXA measurement.

▶ **Radiographic findings**
Increased radiolucency ● Accentuation of tensile and compressive trabeculae in the femoral neck ● Picture-frame vertebrae ● Generally, 30–50% decrease in bone mass needed for radiographic detection ● Bone density scans (DXA, QCT) thus needed for early detection.

▶ **Bone density findings (DXA)**
Bone density as surface value measured in grams per square centimeter at L1–L4 and femoral neck ● Conversion into T-score and Z-score by comparison with age-specific and sex-specific healthy population.
– T-score compares patient with healthy young individuals (30-year-olds).
– Z-score compares patient with age-adjusted healthy population.
World Health Organization (WHO) osteoporosis (1994) criteria for T-scores:
– Normal bone density: T-score up to –1 SD (standard deviation).
– Osteopenia: T-score between –1 and –2.5 SD.
– Osteoporosis: T-score less than –2.5 SD.
– Established osteoporosis: fracture has occurred.
Indications for DXA: Radiographs raise suspicion of osteoporosis ● Distal radial fracture ● Femoral neck fracture ● Vertebral body fracture in the absence of trauma or with minimal trauma ● Cortisone use ● Positive family history ● Smoking.

▶ **Bone density findings (QCT)**
Bone density measured as volume in milligrams per milliliter at L1–L3 ● QCT may be used as an alternative to DXA ● WHO osteoporosis criteria do not apply to QCT.

Fig. 4.1   Osteoporosis in a 66-year-old woman. Lateral radiograph of the lumbar spine. Markedly increased radiolucency and formation of codfish vertebrae involving L1, L2, and L4.

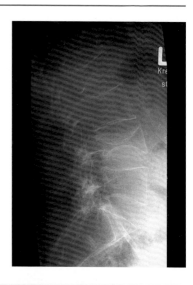

Fig. 4.2   Osteoporosis in a 79-year-old woman. Pelvic radiograph showing increased radiolucency and typical accentuation of tensile and compressive trabeculae.

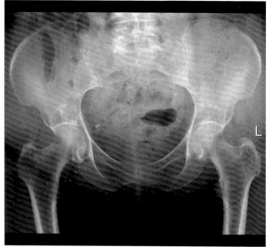

– Normal bone density: calcium hydroxyapatite > 120 mg/ml.
– Osteopenia: calcium hydroxyapatite 80–120 mg/ml.
– Osteoporosis: calcium hydroxyapatite < 80 mg/ml.
▶ **Quantitative sonography findings**
Does not allow quantification of bone density • Cannot replace DXA or QCT scans • DXA recommended in any event.

Clinical Aspects

Early disease is clinically silent • First symptom is usually osteoporotic fracture • Early detection is vital • Fractures typically associated with osteoporosis include distal radial fracture, vertebral body fracture, and femoral neck fracture.
▶ **Treatment options**
Management of osteopenia includes calcium and vitamin D therapy, a diet high in dairy products, and exercise • Treatment of osteoporosis also includes bisphosphonates.
▶ **Course and prognosis**
After fracture, risk of refracture increases 13-fold • Good prognosis if detected early • Bisphosphonates reduce the incidence of fractures after 2 years by 50–70%.
▶ **What does the clinician want to know?**
Fractures • WHO score (T-score) • Signs of secondary osteoporosis • Osteomalacia.

Differential Diagnosis

Osteomalacia	– Blurred appearance of trabeculae
	– Looser transformation zones (radiolucent cortical lines running perpendicular to the cortex/insufficiency fractures)
Renal osteodystrophy	– Subperiosteal resorption in the hand and subchondral areas of resorption
	– Cortical tunneling
	– Increased levels of parathyroid hormone (PTH)
Metastases	– Well-defined osteolytic lesions
	– MRI for differentiation
Multiple myeloma	– Focal lytic lesions or diffuse osteoporosis
	– MRI for differentiation

Tips and Pitfalls

False-negative DXA findings: artificially elevated bone density score, e.g., in patients with aortic sclerosis, spondylosis, spondylarthritis, or osteoma • Pre-existing vertebral body fractures must be ruled out before measurement • Misdiagnosing multiple myeloma as osteoporosis (electrophoresis whenever myeloma is suspected).

Selected References

Blake GM, Fogelmann I. Role of dual-energy X-ray absorptiometry in the diagnosis and treatment of osteoporosis [review]. J Clin Densitom 2007; 10(1): 102–110

Guglielmi G, Perta A, Palladino D, Crisetti N, Mischitelli F, Cammisa M. Bone densitometry in the diagnosis and follow-up of osteoporosis [in Italian]. Radiol Med (Torino) 2003; 106(3 Suppl 1): 29–35

Kanis JA. Diagnosis of osteoporosis and fracture risk. Lancet 2002; 359: 1929–1936

Melton LJ, Chrischilles EA, Cooper C, Lane AW, Riggs BL. How many women have osteoporosis? J Bone Miner Res 1992; 7(9): 1005–1010

Royal College of Physicians. Osteoporosis: clinical guidelines for prevention and treatment. Available at: http://www.rcplondon.ac.uk/pubs/wp/wp_osteo_update.htm. Accessed January 2, 2007

Wagner S, Baur-Melnyk A, Sittek H, et al. Diagnosis of osteoporosis: visual assessment of conventional and digital radiography in comparison with dual X-ray absorptiometry (DEXA) of the lumbar spine. Osteoporos Int 2005; 16(12): 1815–1822

Definition

▶ **Epidemiology**
Formerly affected mainly working-class children ● Rarely seen today ● Twice as common among girls as among boys.

▶ **Etiology, pathophysiology, pathogenesis**
Vitamin D deficiency during growth ● Deficiency leads to undermineralization of bone ● Histology shows predominance of uncalcified osteoid.
Vitamin D is produced in the liver (7-dehydrocholesterol) and transformed in the skin by UV light into cholecalciferol ● Two-step process of hydroxylation in the liver and kidney to form 1,25-dihydroxycholecalciferol (active vitamin D₃) ● Causes: malnutrition ● Inadequate exposure to sunlight ● X-linked hydroxylation defect in the kidney ● End-organ resistance at the bone ● Phosphate diabetes: abnormal resorption of phosphate in proximal renal tubule ● Malabsorption (celiac disease, cystic fibrosis) ● Anticonvulsants.

Imaging Signs

▶ **Modality of choice**
Conventional radiography.

▶ **Pathognomonic findings**
Cupping, disorganized metaphysis with indistinct margins (especially in distal radius) ● Widened epiphyseal plate ● Bowing deformity of extremities.

▶ **Radiographic findings**
Changes are especially apparent in the growth plates of the rapidly growing bones: distal ulna and metaphyses of the knee ● Increased radiolucency due to undermineralization ● Widened epiphyseal plate ● Metaphyseal cupping with indistinct margins ● Enlargement of the costochondral joints ("rachitic rosary") ● Growth retardation ● Bowing deformity of long tubular bones ● Scoliosis ● Three-cornered (distorted, contracted) pelvis ● Basilar impression ● "Slipped" femoral head epiphysis.

Clinical Aspects

▶ **Typical presentation**
Disproportional dwarfism (long trunk relative to short extremities) ● Rachitic rosary ● Craniotabes ● Bowlegs ● Scoliosis ● Poor muscle tone ● Muscle cramps ● Increased susceptibility to infection ● Laboratory tests: hypocalcemia, hypophosphatemia.

▶ **Treatment options**
Depends on cause: UV light therapy ● Vitamin D₃, calcium supplements ● Since breast milk contains little vitamin D, substitution therapy may be considered in babies who are exclusively breastfed.

▶ **Course and prognosis**
Early radiographic changes are usually reversible.

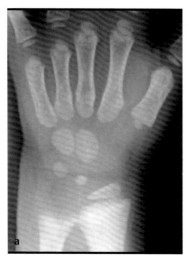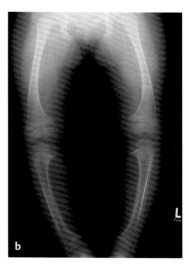

Fig. 4.3 a, b Rickets in a 2-year-old girl.

a Radiograph of the wrist joint showing widening and cupping of the epiphyseal plate in the radius and "fraying" metaphyses.

b Radiograph of both legs showing varus deformity of the lower extremities, widening of the medial epiphyseal plates, and indistinct contours.

▶ **What does the clinician want to know?**
Presence of typical rachitic changes ● Bowing deformities ● Fractures.

Differential Diagnosis
....

Scurvy　　　　　　　　– Sclerotic line in the metaphysis, bordering with
(vitamin C deficiency)　　a radiolucent line
　　　　　　　　　　　　– Sclerotic ring around the epiphysis (Wimberger sign)
　　　　　　　　　　　　– Metaphyseal spurs

Tips and Pitfalls
....

Presentation usually classic ● Failure to consider rickets as a potential diagnosis, given its rarity.

Selected References

Pitt MJ. Rickets and osteomalacia are still around. Radiol Clin North Am 1991; 29(1): 97–118

Wharton B, Bishop N. Rickets. Lancet 2003; 362 (9393): 1389–1400

Definition

▶ **Epidemiology**
Predominantly older patients with vitamin D$_3$ deficiency ● One study found vitamin D deficiency in 60% of patients with femoral neck fracture.

▶ **Etiology, pathophysiology, pathogenesis**
Abnormal bone mineralization in adults due to vitamin D$_3$ deficiency ● Deficiency leads to excessive uncalcified, pathologic osteoid.
  – Vitamin D deficiency: malassimilation syndrome ● Dietary deficiency ● Inadequate exposure to UV light.
  – Abnormal vitamin D metabolism, e.g., liver or renal insufficiency.
  – Secondary to vitamin-D-independent osteomalacia in renal tubular disorders (phosphate diabetes, renal tubular acidosis) ● Phosphatase deficiency.
  – Paraneoplastic ● Association with mesenchymal soft-tissue tumors (hyperphosphaturia).
Vitamin D$_3$ deficiency leads to calcium deficiency which then causes secondary hyperparathyroidism ● This in turn results in increased bone breakdown ● Ultimately bone loss follows ● Results in rickets in children and osteomalacia in adults.

Imaging Signs

▶ **Modality of choice**
Conventional radiographs of thoracic and lumbar spine (lateral) as well as femur and pelvis.

▶ **Pathognomonic findings**
Looser transformation zones ● Bone structure appears blurred ● Increased radiolucency.

▶ **Radiographic findings**
Increased transparency of bone ● Trabeculae appear indistinct (blurred or ground-glass appearance, representing uncalcified osteoid) ● Cortical tunneling in small tubular bones (nonspecific) ● Skeletal deformity in late stages as a sign of static insufficiency of the bone ● Distorted, three-cornered pelvis with protrusio acetabuli ● Kyphoscoliosis ● Bell-shaped thorax ● Bowing deformity of long bones.
Looser transformation zones: Narrow, transverse radiolucent lines in the cortex (consistent with cortical insufficiency fractures caused by stress) ● Virtually no signs of consolidation ● Typically affected are the femora, scapulae, ribs, pubis, and ischial tuberosities ● Multiple Looser zones are referred to as Milkman syndrome.

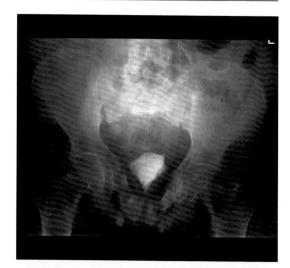

Fig. 4.4 Pelvic radiograph in a 55-year-old woman with severe osteomalacia caused by lack of exposure to sunlight. Blurring of the bone structure and bilateral insufficiency fractures of the pubis and ischial tuberosities as well as pronounced Milkman syndrome.

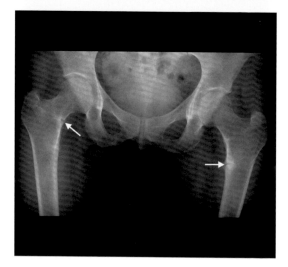

Fig. 4.5 Osteomalacia in a 43-year-old woman. Pelvic radiograph showing typical Looser transformation zones along the medial femoral neck on both sides.

Clinical Aspects

▶ **Typical presentation**
Generalized, diffuse, dull bone pain (periosteal expansion pain from bone deformation), especially in skeletal regions under great stress such as the lumbar spine, pelvis, and legs • Pain also on pressure • Pain • Symptoms of hypocalcemia such as tetany and muscle weakness • Characteristic laboratory findings: hypophosphatemia, elevated alkaline phosphatase, low vitamin D levels.

▶ **Treatment options**
Vitamin D_3 and calcium replacement therapy (1000–1500 mg daily) • Treat any underlying disease (renal or liver insufficiency).

▶ **Course and prognosis**
Good prognosis with vitamin D replacement therapy • Osteoid mineralization with therapy.

▶ **What does the clinician want to know?**
Looser transformation zones • Mineralization (osteopenia?) • Fractures • Skeletal deformities.

Differential Diagnosis

Osteoporosis	– No Looser zones
	– Increased radiolucency, but no blurring of bone structure
Primary hyper-parathyroidism	– Subperiosteal resorption in the hands
	– Brown tumors
	– Osteopenia, but no blurring of bone structure

Selected References

Cooper KL. Radiology of metabolic bone disease [review]. Endocrinol Metab Clin North Am 1989; 18(4): 955–976

Jevtic V. Imaging of renal osteodystrophy [review]. Eur J Radiol 2003; 46(2): 85–95

Schneider R. Radiologic methods of evaluating generalized osteopenia [review]. Orthop Clin North Am 1984; 15(4): 631–651

Definition

Synonym: osteitis fibrosa cystica (von Recklinghausen disease)

▶ **Epidemiology**
Prevalence of 4 in 100 000 ● Women affected twice as often as men.

▶ **Etiology, pathophysiology, pathogenesis**
Primary hyperparathyroidism: Autonomous hyperfunction of the parathyroid gland (85% solitary, 15% multiple adenomas), hyperplasia, or carcinoma ● Increased familial incidence associated with multiple endocrine neoplasias (MEN1 or MEN2) ● Autonomous excessive production of parathormone ● Overproduction leads to high calcium resorption from the bones.
Secondary hyperparathyroidism: Long-term hypocalcemia in vitamin D_3 deficiency, e.g., due to chronic renal insufficiency or malabsorption ● Parathyroid hyperplasia.
Tertiary hyperparathyroidism: Development of autonomous adenoma of parathyroid glands in long-standing secondary hyperparathyroidism.

Imaging Signs

▶ **Modality of choice**
Conventional radiography (especially of the hands).

▶ **Pathognomonic findings**
Typical changes in the hands: subperiosteal resorption on the radial aspects ● Cortical tunneling ● Brown tumors.

▶ **Radiographic findings**
Signs of increased breakdown of bone consistent with osteoporosis.
– Subperiosteal resorption: irregular, superficial cortical defects ● Predilection for radial aspects of phalanges, also femoral neck, proximal humerus, proximal tibia, ribs, submarginal along joints (acromioclavicular joint, sternoclavicular joint, SI joint, pubic symphysis).
– Intracortical resorption: tunneling/fraying of phalangeal cortices ● Subtendinous resorption at sites under mechanical stress (e.g., patella, calcaneus).
– Subchondral resorption: thinning of subchondral bone end plate at joints.
– Brown tumors: circumscribed areas of bone lysis (especially facial bones, pelvis, ribs, and femur).
– Chondrocalcinosis: sclerotic radiodense bands near the vertebral end plates.
Resorption reversible with therapy ● Brown tumors calcify and over the years are replaced by lamellar bone.

▶ **MRI findings**
Brown tumors: appear on fat-saturated T2-weighted images as focal structures that are isointense to fluid ● There may be fluid–fluid levels due to hemorrhage.

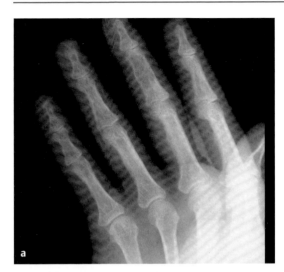

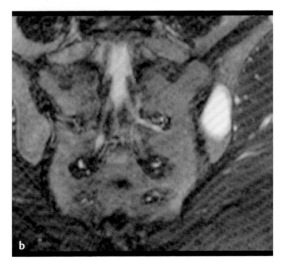

Fig. 4.6 a, b
Primary hyperparathyroidism in a 28-year-old woman.
a Radiograph of the hand. Intracortical resorption (cortical tunneling), osteopenia, and subperiosteal resorption, predominantly affecting the proximal and middle phalanges of the third and fourth fingers. Brown tumor on the middle phalanx of the third finger.
b Fat-saturated paracoronal MRI of the sacrum. Brown tumor in left ilium showing typical cyst-like signal intensity.

Clinical Aspects

▶ **Typical presentation**
Mnemonic: stones (kidney stones), bones (osseous changes), and groans (stomach ulcers).

▶ **Treatment options**
Primary hyperparathyroidism: resection • Secondary hyperparathyroidism: vitamin D therapy.

▶ **Course and prognosis**
Curable.

▶ **What does the clinician want to know?**
Findings typical of hyperparathyroidism • Differentiation from rheumatoid arthritis.

Differential Diagnosis

Rheumatoid arthritis	– Primarily affects PIP and MCP joints
	– Joint space narrowing
	– Subchondral erosions
	– Synovitis (detectable on MRI)
Ankylosing spondylarthritis	– Mixed picture (erosions, sclerosis) in SI joints
	– Syndesmophytes on the spinal column
Osteoporosis	– Absence of specific signs such as subperiosteal resorption

Tips and Pitfalls

Misdiagnosis as osteoporosis.

Selected References

Johnson NA, Tublin ME, Ogilvie JB. Parathyroid imaging: technique and role in the preoperative evaluation of primary hyperparathyroidism [review]. AJR Am J Roentgenol 2007; 188(6): 1706–1715

Silverberg SJ, Bilezikian JP. The diagnosis and management of asymptomatic primary hyperparathyroidism [review]. Nat Clin Pract Endocrinol Metab 2006; 2(9): 494–503

Silverberg SJ, Shane E, de la Cruz L, et al. Skeletal disease in primary hyperparathyroidism. J Bone Miner Res 1989; 4(3): 283–291

Weber AL, Randolph G, Aksoy FG. The thyroid and parathyroid glands. CT and MR imaging and correlation with pathology and clinical findings [review]. Radiol Clin North Am 2000; 38(5): 1105–1129

Definition

▶ **Epidemiology**
Growth disorder involving the volar ulnar radial epiphysis ● Deviation of the hand toward the radius ● Distally prominent ulna (bayonet deformity) ● More common among adolescent girls ● Associated with Turner syndrome ● Bilateral in 50%.

▶ **Etiology, pathophysiology, pathogenesis**
Classification by Henry and Thornburn:
  – Post-traumatic after repetitive microtrauma ● After a single trauma event with abnormal healing of volar ulnar radial epiphysis.
  – Dysplastic ● Associated with bone dysplasias such as osteochondromatosis, Ollier disease, achondroplasia, mucopolysaccharidosis.
  – Chromosomal anomalies (X-linked mutation, Turner syndrome).
  – Idiopathic.

Imaging Signs

▶ **Modality of choice**
Radiographs in two planes.

▶ **Radiographic findings**
Relevant features affecting articulation of the distal radial articular surface:
  – Increased inclination of the radial articular surface toward the ulna: widened angle between the distal radial articular surface and a perpendicular line to the long axis of the radius, measured on a PA view (normal range: 21–23°).
  – Volar tilt: increased angle between the distal radial articular surface and a line perpendicular to the long axis of the radius, measured on a lateral view (normal range: 10–15°).
  – Radial and dorsal curvature of the distal radius.
  – Shortened radius ● Ulna appears longer than radius.
  – Joint incongruence ● Possible incongruence of distal radioulnar joint.
  – Premature closure of epiphyseal plate on the ulnar side of the distal radius.
  – Focal osteopenia on the ulnar side of the distal radius.
  – Triangular (teardrop-shaped) deformity of the distal radial epiphysis and V-shaped configuration of the proximal carpus.
  – Exostosis on the distal ulnar radius.
  – Relative dorsal subluxation of ulna compared to the radius and carpal bones or palmar subluxation of carpal bones.

▶ **CT findings**
If necessary, obtain CT scan for three-dimensional imaging of the deformity.

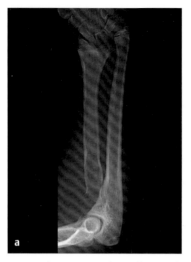 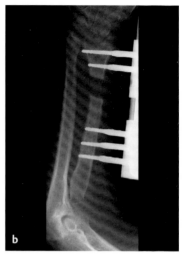

Fig. 5.1 a, b Forearm radiographs in Madelung deformity.
a Shortened radius and V-shaped configuration of the carpal bones.
b Follow-up radiograph. Callus distraction of the radius.

Clinical Aspects

► **Typical presentation**

Shortened and malaligned radius (bayonet deformity) ● Radial club hand in patients with severe deformity ● Deformity worsens progressively until growth stops ● Progressive deformity is associated with increasing pain and decreasing range of motion ● Supination and dorsiflexion are especially affected.

► **Treatment options**

Depend on patient age, severity of deformity, clinical symptoms, and radiological findings.

– Vicker physiolysis: when deformity is detected before cessation of growth ● Ulnar-volar release with partial resection of affected epiphysis ● Only a portion of the epiphysis is preserved ● Stimulates compensatory growth.

– Radial osteotomy: when deformity is detected late ● Usually corrective osteotomy of the radius to re-establish adequate articulation at the distal radio-ulnar joint ● In marked ulna-plus variance, ulnar shortening osteotomy is also an option ● Alternative method: distraction of the radius using the Ilizarov technique.

– Resection of the distal ulnar head (to restore rotation).

– Wrist arthrodesis for treatment of pronounced secondary degenerative changes.

▶ **Course and prognosis**
Progressive subluxation until cessation of growth ● Relatively good postoperative outcome ● Range of motion may nevertheless be limited.

▶ **What does the clinician want to know?**
Extent of deformity (volar and radial tilt) ● Stage of growth plate closure.

Tips and Pitfalls
....

Discreet signs may be missed.

Selected References

Anton JI, Reitz GB, Spiegel MB. Madelung's deformity. Ann Surg 1938; 108(3): 411–439

De Billy B, Gastaud F, Repetto M. Treatment of Madelung's deformity by lengthening and reaxation of the distal extremity of the radius by Ilizarov's technique. Eur J Pediatr Surg 1994; 7: 296–298

Felman AH, Kirkpatrick JA Jr. Madelung's deformity: observations in 17 patients. Radiology 1969; 93(5): 1037–1042

Schwartz RP, Sumner TE. Madelung's deformity as a presenting sign of Turner's syndrome. J Pediatr 2000; 136(4): 563

Villeco J. Case report and review of the literature: Madelung's deformity. J Hand Ther 2002; 15(4): 355–362

Developmental Disorders

Definition

▶ **Epidemiology**
Most common congenital developmental abnormality of the skeletal system (abnormal acetabular development) • Incidence varies regionally • 2–4% in Western Europe • Girls are affected six times as often as boys.

▶ **Etiology, pathophysiology, pathogenesis**
Multifactorial etiology with endogenous and exogenous factors • Risk factors: breech presentation, familial incidence, premature birth, female sex • Secondary in connective tissue diseases such as Ehlers–Danlos syndrome.
Primary cause is abnormal ossification of the acetabular rim with possible cartilage deformity (more vertically oriented, shallow, and cranially elongated acetabulum) • If untreated, the femoral head may become decentered leading to subluxation, dislocation, or even development of a secondary acetabulum (prearthritic deformity) • Often delayed ossification of the femoral head ossification center on the affected side • Secondary deformity of the femoral neck (coxa valga and anteversion) possible.

Imaging Signs

▶ **Modality of choice**
Radiographs (AP pelvic view, usually during toddler stage, after clinical or sonographic suspicion of dysplasia) • Sonography (primary examination modality in infants) • Possibly MRI • Direct MR/CT arthrography studies in adult patients if needed.

▶ **Radiographic findings**
Pelvic radiograph: Delayed ossification of epiphyseal ossification center and instability (ossification of epiphyseal ossific nucleus begins in the 2nd month or later).
Acetabular roof angle after Hilgenreiner (acetabular index): Angle between the Hilgenreiner line (imaginary horizontal line between the triradiate cartilages of the acetabula; Y-line) and a line from the superolateral to the inferomedial end of the acetabular margin • 30° at birth • 20° in school-age children • Angle > 30° is a sign of hip dysplasia.
Reimer index: Femoral head is divided into two parts by the Perkin–Ombrédanne line (running perpendicular from the acetabular rim to the Hilgenreiner line) • Reimer migration index = horizontal diameter of the lateral part of the femur as a percentage of the diameter of the entire epiphyseal ossification center • Normal > 20% • If < 20%, the femoral head is lateralized • In hip dislocation, flexion and external rotation views may be useful to check reduction potential.

▶ **CT findings**
Useful in assessing complicated dislocations • Measurement of femoral and acetabular anteversion • Better visualization of bone blocks after dislocation.

▶ **MRI findings**
Preoperative and postoperative evaluation of complex dislocations • Assessment of reduction outcome, labrum, capsule, and acetabular cartilage • Surveillance of postoperative complications, e.g., femoral head necrosis.

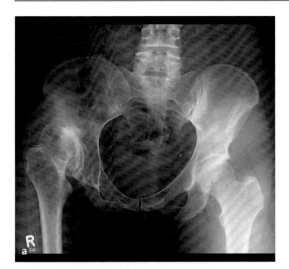

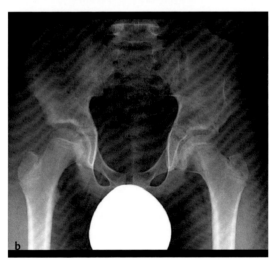

Fig. 5.2 a, b Pelvic radiograph in right-sided hip dysplasia. **a** Vertically oriented acetabulum which is elongated cranially (formation of a secondary acetabulum). Widened femoral head with external rotation (lesser trochanter is fully visible) and increased valgus position. **b** Good surgical result after pelvic osteotomy. The left femoral head is centered in the acetabulum with only minimal deformity.

Fig. 5.3 Radio-
graphic lines of the
pelvis for assessing
hip dysplasia.

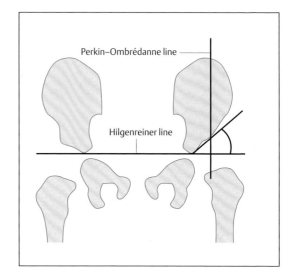

Perkin–Ombrédanne line

Hilgenreiner line

Clinical Aspects

▸ **Typical presentation**
Restricted range of motion (limited abduction) • Asymmetrical skin folds • Un-
equal leg lengths • Ortolani sign.

▸ **Treatment options**
Conservative: Brace or harness • Closed reduction • Orthosis/cast.
Operative: Surgical reduction • Corrective pelvic osteotomy (acetabuloplasty,
Salter osteotomy, triple osteotomy, Chiari pelvic osteotomy) • Corrective osteot-
omy of the proximal femur.

▸ **Course and prognosis**
The earlier treatment begins, the better the prognosis • In patients with established (sub-)luxation, prognosis depends on achieving a stable, centered hip and
stable acetabular roof over the femoral head • Complications: redislocation, secondary osteoarthritis, femoral head necrosis.

▸ **What does the clinician want to know?**
Disease stage • Follow-up.

Tips and Pitfalls

Radiographic assessment of only one hip.

Selected References

Dillon JE, Connolly SA, Connolly LP, Kim YJ, Jaramillo D. MR imaging of congenital/developmental and acquired disorders of the pediatric hip and pelvis. Magn Reson Imaging Clin North Am 2005; 13(4): 783–797

Harcke HT. Imaging methods used for children with hip dysplasia. Clin Orthop Relat Res 2005; (434): 71–77

Marega L. The management of version abnormalities and angular deformities in developmental dysplasia of the hip. Orthopedics 2005; 28(9 Suppl): s1097–1099

Smergel E, Losik SB, Rosenberg HK. Sonography of hip dysplasia. Ultrasound Q 2004; 20(4): 201–216

Woolacott NF, Puhan MA, Steurer J, Kleijnen J. Ultrasonography in screening for developmental dysplasia of the hip in newborns: review. BMJ 2005; 330(7505): 1413

Definition

▶ **Epidemiology**
Growth disorder of unknown cause ● Mainly affects the medial portion of the proximal tibial epiphysis and medial portions of the metaphysis and epiphysis ● Leads to varus deformity ● Usually bilateral involvement (80% in infantile and 50% in late-onset disease), less often unilateral ● Increased incidence among black children in South Africa and Jamaica.

▶ **Etiology, pathophysiology, pathogenesis**
Etiology unclear ● Possibly due to abnormal stress on the posteromedial proximal tibial epiphysis ● Risk factors: early walking, obesity, black family (earlier walking) ● Slight displacement of the medial tibial epiphysis lateralward ● Growth disturbance affecting the medial portion of the epiphysis ● Compression of the medial metaphysis. ● Varus deformity progresses with growth.
Three types:
- Infantile tibia vara: usually bilateral ● Age 1–3.5 years ● Most common type ● Severe disease course.
- Juvenile tibia vara: age 4–10 years.
- Adolescent tibia vara: usually unilateral ● Age 10–15 years.
The latter two types are occasionally the result of previously undetected infantile tibia vara.

Imaging Signs

▶ **Modality of choice**
Radiography (AP standing views of the knee) ● Possibly MRI.

▶ **Radiographic findings**
Depression of the medial tibial epiphysis ● "Beaking" ● Varus deformity of the tibia.
Six stages classified by Langenskiold (to guide prognosis and treatment):
- Stage I: Varus deformity of the tibia with concomitant irregular growth plate ● Small "beak" on the medial aspect of the metaphysis ● Age 2–3 years.
- Stage II: Evidence of depression of the medial metaphysis ● Angulation of the medial epiphysis ● Age 2–4 years.
- Stage III: Progressive varus deformity ● Prominent "beak" ● There may be fragmentation of the medial metaphysis ● Age 4–6 years.
- Stage IV: Distinctly narrowed growth plate ● Strong angulation of the medial epiphysis (irregular border) ● Age 5–10 years.
- Stage V: Marked deformity of the medial epiphysis, which is now divided into two parts by a clearly visible band (distal part: triangular) ● Age 9–11 years.
- Stage VI: Bony bridge between the epiphysis and metaphysis ● There may be fusion of the triangular fragment of the separated portion of the epiphysis with the metaphysis ● Age 10–13 years.
Irreparable structural damage in stages V and VI.

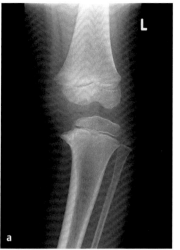 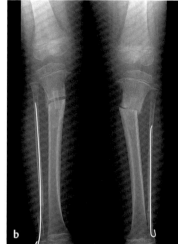

Fig. 5.4 a, b Blount disease.
a AP standing radiograph of the left knee. Spur formation on the medial metaphysis of the tibia, varus deformity of the proximal tibia and thus varus malalignment of the knee.
b AP view of both lower legs and knee joints. Follow-up radiograph after proximal corrective osteotomy of the tibia and intramedullary nailing of the fibula. The axis of the knee joint has been restored.

▶ **CT findings**
  Coronally reconstructed CT images are occasionally helpful for assessment of the epiphyseal plate.
▶ **MRI findings**
  Early-stage diagnosis ● Evaluation of epiphyseal plate and epiphysis.

Developmental Disorders

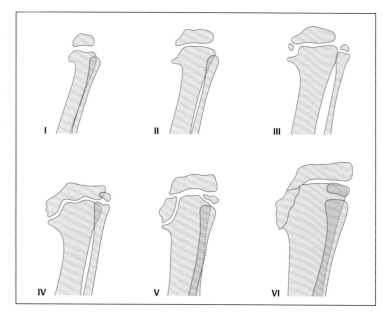

Fig. 5.5 Stages of progression in Blount disease.

Clinical Aspects

▶ **Typical presentation**
Symptoms begin with limping during the second year of life (infantile type) or between the ages of 6 and 12 (juvenile form) ● Varus knee ● Distal femur not affected ● Leg-length discrepancy in unilateral or asymmetrical disease ● Medial tibial metaphysis occasionally palpable.

▶ **Treatment options**
Conservative: Orthotic braces.
Surgical: If deformity advances despite attempted conservative treatment: valgus-producing high tibial osteotomy ● In patients with fusion of the epiphyseal plate, resection of the bony bridge and epiphysiodesis in addition to osteotomy.

▶ **Course and prognosis**
If left untreated, deformity progresses and is potentially irreparable.

▶ **What does the clinician want to know?**
Disease stage ● Rule out differential diagnoses.

Differential Diagnosis

Rickets	– Widening of the growth plate – Affected region usually shows cupping with indistinct margins – No ossification of the metaphyses
Physiologic bowing	– Normal growth plates – No depression of the medial tibial epiphysis – No "beaking"
Tibial plateau fracture	– No "beaking" – Often lateral involvement – Patient history
Osteomyelitis	– Occasionally difficult to distinguish – Typical MRI findings – Patient history
Ollier disease	– Enchondroma: typical findings on radiographic and MRI studies
Metaphyseal skeletal dysplasias	– Always symmetrical
Focal fibrocartilaginous dysplasia	– Always unilateral – Characteristic defect on medial tibial metaphyseal cortex

Tips and Pitfalls

Mistaking disease for physiologic bowing.

Selected References

Bradway JK, Klassen RA, Peterson HA. Blount disease: a review of the English literature. J Pediatr Orthop 1987; 7(4): 472–480

Cheema JI, Grissom LE, Harcke HT. Radiographic characteristics of lower-extremity bowing in children. Radiographics 2003; 23(4): 871–880

Definition

▶ **Epidemiology**
Prepubescence and early adolescence • Epiphyseal separation at the proximal end of the femur and displacement of the femoral head, usually posteromedially and inferiorly • Incidence is 2 in 100 000 youths under age 20 • Boys affected 2–3 times as often as girls • Bilateral in up to 50% • Peak incidence in girls is at age 12 and in boys at age 14 • Increased familial incidence in 5–10% of cases.

▶ **Etiology, pathophysiology, pathogenesis**
Mixed etiology: Hormonal factors • Growth spurt • Physical activity • Obesity • Damage arising from toxicity • May also occur after chemotherapy or radiation treatment • Family history.
(Pre-)pubertal widening and reorientation of the physeal cartilage • Diminished mechanical resistance (overload due to obesity or intense athletic activity) • Increased shear forces due to angular (in contrast to horizontal) orientation • Abductors pull the femur anteriorly and laterally: the epiphysis remains in the acetabulum, but is tilted medially and posteriorly relative to the femoral neck • Salter–Harris type I fracture.

Imaging Signs

▶ **Modality of choice**
Radiographs of both hips in AP and axial views (after Lauenstein) • Perhaps MRI.

▶ **Radiographic findings**
AP: Widening of the epiphyseal plate • Appearance of epiphyseal narrowing due to posterior tilt • A line drawn tangential to the superolateral femoral neck will not intersect the epiphysis.
Axial: Direct visualization of tilting • Measurement of degree of slippage: angle between a line drawn perpendicular to the tangent to the femoral neck and the intersections of the physis with the cortex • Prognostic indicator of long-term joint degeneration.
Remodeling changes in chronic disease: Rounding off of the metaphysis • Defect filling in the physis.

▶ **MRI findings**
Earlier detection of physeal changes than on conventional radiographs • Widening and increased signal intensity on T2-weighted images • Bone marrow edema may be present • Helpful study when diagnosis is difficult, if there is clinical suspicion despite unremarkable radiographic findings, or to check contralateral side • Modality of choice in femoral head necrosis (up to 18% in acute disease).

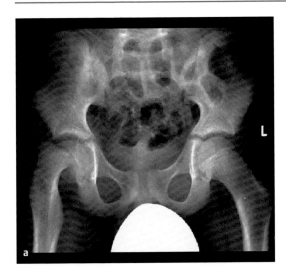

Fig. 5.6 a, b Slipped capital femoral epiphysis (SCFE). Acute slippage on the right side with risk of femoral head necrosis due to disrupted blood supply and incipient slippage on the left side.
a Pelvic radiograph.
b Pelvic radiograph (axial view) of the right hip joint.

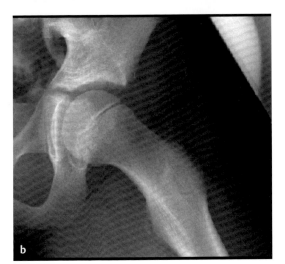

Fig. 5.7 a–c This patient had pain and antalgic gait for several weeks during athletic activity. **a** Pelvic radiograph showing widened and blurry appearance of the left epiphyseal plate compared to the right side.

b Radiograph of the left hip joint (axial view) showing remodeling of the proximal metaphysis. Considerable posteroinferior slippage of the femoral head and incipient sclerosis are already present.

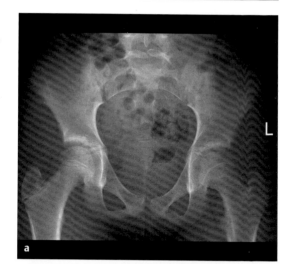

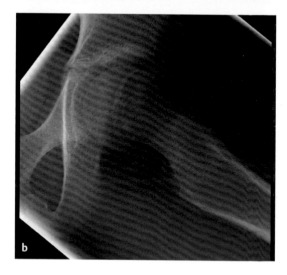

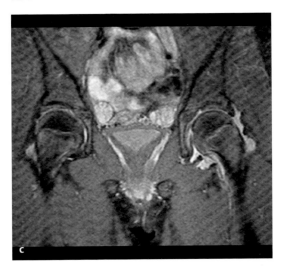

c MRI. Coronal fat-saturated T2-weighted image showing slipped femoral head.

Clinical Aspects

▶ **Typical presentation**

Hip and knee pain ● Limping ● Often limited internal rotation at the hip joint ● Sometimes also restricted abduction.

- Imminent slipped capital femoral epiphysis: presence of typical symptoms without radiological evidence of slippage.
- Acute slipped capital femoral epiphysis: symptoms for less than 2 weeks with imminent increased slippage. Acute form can develop as a sudden progression of chronic disease.
- Chronic slipped capital femoral epiphysis: symptoms persist for more than 2 weeks; slippage occurs slowly and may last for several months.

Classified by walking ability: stable (= ambulatory patient), unstable (= nonambulatory patient).

▶ **Treatment options**

Full-blown stage: operative management is essential in acute and chronic forms ● In pediatric orthopedics, acute epiphyseal slippage is an indication for emergency surgery ● Surgical fixation (pin or screw fixation, corrective osteotomy) ● Complications: chondrolysis, femoral head necrosis, premature physeal closure, infection, screw/nail breakage ● Preventive stabilization of the contralateral side is usual.

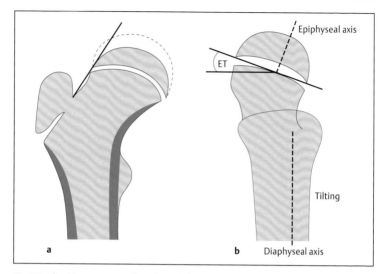

Fig. 5.8 a, b Measurement of epiphyseal slip angle.
a AP projection. Tangent drawn to the superior border of the femoral neck does not intersect the epiphysis.
b Axial projection. The axes of the femoral neck and epiphysis are no longer parallel (NB: because of projection, deviations up to 10° on radiographs should not be considered as certain signs of pathology) and a slip angle or epiphyseal torsion angle (ET) is seen. The angle of slippage is determined by a line drawn tangential to the femoral neck and a line perpendicular to the epiphyseal axis.

▶ **Course and prognosis**
Acute slippage: spontaneous stabilization is unlikely ● Chronic slippage: self-limiting due to physeal ossification, seating of femoral head on femoral neck, and ossification of the fibrocartilage ring ● In 40% of cases there is also slippage on the contralateral side ● Increased risk of early osteoarthritis and femoral head necrosis.

▶ **What does the clinician want to know?**
Diagnosis ● Degree of tilt ● Complications.

Differential Diagnosis

Septic coxitis	– Clinical signs and symptoms – No slippage – Effusion
Hip dysplasia	– Normal-appearing physis – No slippage – Characteristic acetabular deformity
Perthes' disease	– Younger age group – Deformed epiphyseal ossification center

Tips and Pitfalls

Missing or underestimating the importance of very slight findings.

Selected References

Ducou Le Pointe H, Sirinelli D. Limb emergencies in children. J Radiol 2005; 86(2 Pt 2): 237–249

Hell AK. Slipped capital femoral epiphysis and overweight. Orthopäde 2005; 34(7): 658–663

Liu SC, Tsai CC, Huang CH. Atypical slipped capital femoral epiphysis after radiotherapy and chemotherapy. Clin Orthop Relat Res 2004; (426): 212–218

Parsch K, Zehender H, Buhl T, Weller S. Intertrochanteric corrective osteotomy for moderate and severe chronic slipped capital femoral epiphysis. J Pediatr Orthop B 1999; 8(3): 223–230

Reynolds RA. Diagnosis and treatment of slipped capital femoral epiphysis. Curr Opin Pediatr 1999; 11(1): 80–83

Uglow MG, Clarke NM. The management of slipped capital femoral epiphysis. J Bone Joint Surg Br 2004; 86(5): 631–635

Definition

▶ **Epidemiology**
Congenital foot deformity with fixed plantar flexion and varus heel, and adduction and supination of the forefoot ● Incidence: 1.2–2.3 per 1000 live births ● Boys affected twice as often as girls.

▶ **Etiology, pathophysiology, pathogenesis**
Genetic factors (polygenic) ● Environmental factors during pregnancy ● Primary deformity is medial deviation of talar neck or fibromatosis affecting the deltoid ligament ● Classification: congenital club foot, positional club foot, congenital talipes varus, neurogenic club foot, and club foot deformity in arthrogryposis.

Imaging Signs

▶ **Modality of choice**
Radiographs in two planes (DP and lateral views) ● Radiographs are not taken at birth, but during splintage at 4 months for possible surgical indication and operative planning ● Views of the foot in maximum dorsiflexion (assessment of Achilles tendon shortening).

▶ **Radiographic findings**
Views of the foot in corrective position ● Talocalcaneal angle on DP views < 15° (normal: 15–40°) and lateral views < 25° (normal: 25–45°) ● Subluxation of navicular bone (DP projection) ● Ossific nuclei in the talus, calcaneus, cuboid, and metatarsal bones are already radiographically visible at birth ● Ossific nucleus is undetectable in the navicular (which ossifies during the 3rd year of life), complicating accurate assessment of talonavicular subluxation ● Information on the position of the navicular may be derived from the angle between the axis of the talus and the first metatarsal bone ● Tibiocalcaneal angle on lateral radiographs > 90° (normal: 60–90°) ● Calcaneus declines from posterior to anterior ● Adduction deformity: on DP projections the axis through the talus runs lateral to the base of the first metatarsal.

Clinical Aspects

▶ **Typical presentation**
Palpable prominent anterior end of the talus ● Thin skin with tiny creases in this region ● Shortened Achilles tendon, palpable as a tough cord ● Lateral malleolus is displaced posteriorly ● Small high heel ● Thin calves.

▶ **Treatment options**
Four stages of treatment in severe club foot deformity:
  – Stage I: Manipulation and casting (beginning immediately after birth).
  – Stage II: Surgical peritalar release (age 4–6 months).
  – Stage III: Splintage (if forefoot adduction persists).
  – Stage IV: Correction of recurrent deformity and late malalignment problems.

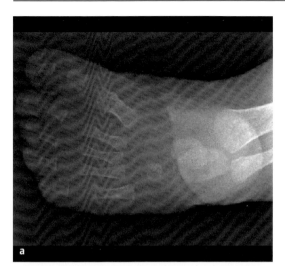

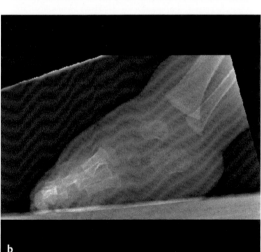

Fig. 5.9 a, b Club foot deformity in a 5-month-old.
a DP radiograph of the foot demonstrates a shortened Achilles tendon, absence of calcaneal inclination from posteroinferior to anterosuperior, and a horizontal talus, producing a diminished talocalcaneal angle.
b Lateral radiograph of the foot. Adduction of the forefoot (axis of the talus is lateral to the first metatarsal) and decreased talocalcaneal angle.

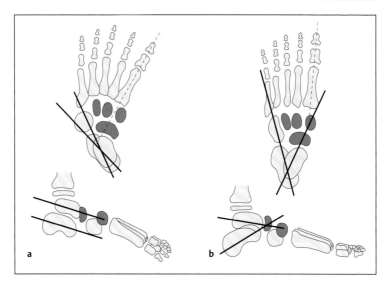

Fig. 5.10 a, b   Measurement of angles in the pediatric foot.
a Construction of the axes through the bisector of the two largest distances of the borders of the ossific nuclei. If the axis of the talus passes lateral to the first metatarsal on a DP radiograph, this is considered a sign of forefoot adduction.
b Normal finding.

Postural club foot is sufficiently treated by manipulation and casting (stage I) ●
Uncomplicated club foot deformities may be adequately managed by stage I and II treatment.

▶ **Course and prognosis**
Deformity that responds well to initial manipulation and casting has a more favorable prognosis ● Degree of calf atrophy correlates with resistance to treatment.

▶ **What does the clinician want to know?**
Progress of initial corrective treatment (stage I, manipulation and casting) and position of ossific nuclei.

Differential Diagnosis

Flatfoot deformity	– Increased talocalcaneal angle (DP view) due to steeply angled talus, subluxating plantarward

Tips and Pitfalls

Taking radiographs with inadequate dorsiflexion of the foot at the ankle joint.

Selected References

Roye DP Jr, Roye BD. Idiopathic congenital talipes equinovarus. J Am Acad Orthop Surg 2002; 10(4): 239–248

Silvani SH. Congenital convex pes valgus. The condition and its treatment. Clin Podiatr Med Surg 1987; 4(1): 163–173

Definition

▶ **Epidemiology**

Incidence of idiopathic scoliosis is 4.5% ● Affects women 1.25 times as often as men ● Proportion of women affected by severe scoliosis is significantly higher.

▶ **Etiology, pathophysiology, pathogenesis**

Idiopathic scoliosis: 70–80% ● Grouped by age of onset: infantile (under 4 years of age), juvenile (4–9 years) and adolescent (10 years to skeletal maturity, 85%).

Secondary scoliosis: In neuromuscular disease and disorders of the nervous system (poliomyelitis, spastic cerebral palsy, syringomyelia, muscular dystrophy), vertebral malformation (e.g., wedge-shaped or hemivertebrae), segmental abnormalities (unilateral or bilateral vertebral fusion), and various other disorders such as neurofibromatosis, achondroplasia, or osteogenesis imperfecta.

Imaging Signs

▶ **Modality of choice**

Radiographs (AP views) of the spine and iliac crests to assess skeletal maturity (ossification of iliac apophysis) ● Any leg-length discrepancies must be adjusted prior to examination.

▶ **Radiographic findings**

Lateral curvature of the vertebral column in the frontal plane.

Evaluation of degree of scoliosis, rotational components, and skeletal maturity.

Scoliosis: Classification based on Cobb angle:

Grade 1: less than 20°

Grade 2: 21–30°

Grade 3: 31–50°

Grade 4: 51–75°

Grade 5: 76–100°

Grade 6: 101–125°

Grade 7: greater than 125°

Rotational components: Pedicle method (Moe method).

Skeletal maturity: Estimation of skeletal maturity: assessment of ossification of the iliac crest apophyses (Risser grades 0–5).

▶ **MRI findings**

Useful for certain diagnoses, e.g., spina bifida, syrinx, meningomyelocele, nerve root anomalies, displacement of the spinal cord/dural sac or "tethered cord."

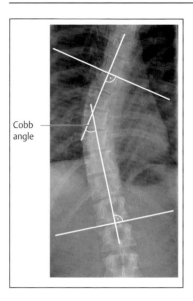

Fig. 5.11   A 16-year-old girl with idiopathic adolescent scoliosis. Right thoracic scoliosis with a Cobb angle of 32°.

Cobb angle

Clinical Aspects

▶ **Typical presentation**
  Scoliosis is usually painless ● Rib humps and lumbar prominence on the convex side of the curvature may be seen on forward bending of the upper body ● Disproportion with shorter trunk.

▶ **Treatment options**
  Treatment determined by Cobb angle: physical therapy if less than 20°, supplemental bracing if 20–50°, and spine-straightening surgery if greater than 50°.

▶ **Course and prognosis**
  Depends on underlying disease and onset of scoliosis ● The earlier the onset, the less favorable the prognosis ● Follow-up evaluation every 6 months is essential ● Along with esthetic and psychosocial problems, severe thoracic scoliosis can also restrict lung function, limiting vital capacity and leading to cor pulmonale.

▶ **What does the clinician want to know?**
  Position of curvature ● Cobb angle ● Changing Cobb angle in the course of disease ● Rotational malalignment ● Additional abnormalities ● Skeletal maturity.

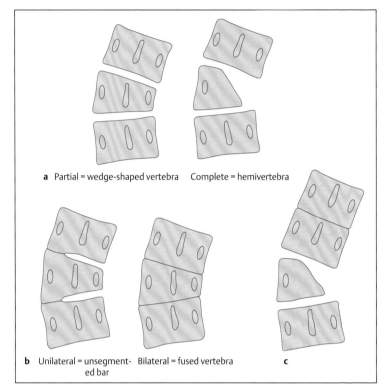

a Partial = wedge-shaped vertebra   Complete = hemivertebra

b Unilateral = unsegment- Bilateral = fused vertebra   **c**
ed bar

Fig. 5.12 a–c Defects of **a** vertebral formation and **b** segmentation. **c** Mixed defect with fused vertebrae and hemivertebra.

Differential Diagnosis

Postural scoliosis   – Curvature in the frontal plane, as in scoliosis, but without vertebral rotation

Tips and Pitfalls

Missing vertebral formation or segmentation defects • Inaccurately estimating the degree of ossification of the iliac crest apophysis (Risser grade) – ossification begins around age 12 and progresses from lateral to medial.

Developmental Disorders

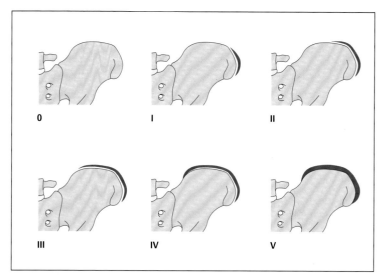

Fig. 5.13 Estimating skeletal age using the Risser method of assessing the iliac crest apophysis.

Selected References

Barnes PD, Brody JD, Jaramillo D, Akbar JU, Emans JB. Atypical idiopathic scoliosis: MR imaging evaluation. Radiology 1993; 186(1): 247–253

Geijer H, Beckman K, Jonsson B, Andersson T, Persliden J. Digital radiography of scoliosis with a scanning method: initial evaluation. Radiology 2001; 218(2): 402–410

Geijer H, Verdonck B, Beckman KW, Andersson T, Persliden J. Digital radiography of scoliosis with a scanning method: radiation dose optimization. Eur Radiol 2003; 13(3): 543–551

Reamy BV, Slakey JB. Adolescent idiopathic scoliosis: review and current concepts. Am Fam Physician 2001; 64(1): 111–116

Definition

▶ **Epidemiology**
Incidence of 1 in 10 000 • Affects men more often than women.

▶ **Etiology, pathophysiology, pathogenesis**
Autosomal dominant inheritance is most common causal factor (more than 150 known mutations), or else new mutations • Sillence classification of four types with varying genetic and phenotypic severity • Underlying cause is abnormal type I collagen.

Imaging Signs

▶ **Modality of choice**
Radiographs of lumbar spine, pelvis, and femur

▶ **Pathognomonic findings**
Generalized osteoporosis • Multiple older fractures • Bowing deformities. • Multiple codfish vertebrae.

▶ **Radiographic findings**
Generalized osteoporosis with increased fragility of the bone • Vertebral body fracture (codfish vertebrae in lumbar spine and wedge-shaped vertebrae in thoracic spine) • Cortical thinning • Bone deformities (contracted pelvis, protrusio acetabuli) • Metaphyseal flaring, sometimes with "cystic" appearance • Kyphoscoliosis (due to ligament laxity and osteoporosis) • Cranium: multiple wormian bones.

Clinical Aspects

▶ **Typical presentation**
Diagnosis is definitive when two of the following four criteria are met:
 – Osteoporosis with abnormal osseous fragility.
 – Blue sclera.
 – Dental enamel anomalies.
 – Presenile hearing loss caused by otosclerosis.

▶ **Treatment options**
Bisphosphonates • Corrective osteotomy to treat deformities.

▶ **Course and prognosis**
Infantile form associated with high fatality rate during infancy and childhood • Osteogenesis imperfecta tarda carries a nearly normal life expectancy.

▶ **What does the clinician want to know?**
Presence of deformities • Fractures.

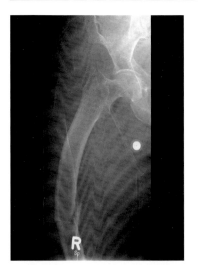

Fig. 5.14 Adult form of osteogenesis imperfecta in a 63-year-old woman. Radiograph of the right femur. Increased radiolucency consistent with osteoporosis. Varus deformity of the femur. Fracture in the middle of the femoral shaft following minor trauma.

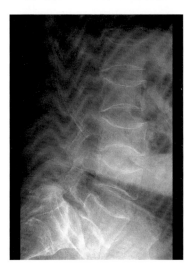

Fig. 5.15 Adult form of osteogenesis imperfecta in a 68-year-old man. Radiograph of the lumbar spine showing typical codfish vertebrae present throughout the entire lumbar spine due to osteoporosis.

Differential Diagnosis

Child abuse	– Patient history
	– No osteoporosis
	– Subperiosteal hemorrhage
	– No blue sclera, no dental anomalies, no kyphoscoliosis
Rickets	– Widened, disorganized growth plates

Tips and Pitfalls

Mild forms frequently misdiagnosed as idiopathic osteoporosis, hence careful inspection of sclera and teeth is warranted.

Selected References

Ablin DS. Osteogenesis imperfecta: a review. Can Assoc Radiol J 1998; 49(2): 110–123

Rauch F, Glorieux FH. Osteogenesis imperfecta [review]. Lancet 2004; 363(9418): 1377–1385

Definition

▶ **Epidemiology**
Bone proliferation disorder ● Incidence of 1 in 20 000–40 000 ● No sex predilection.

▶ **Etiology, pathophysiology, pathogenesis**
Autosomal recessive or autosomal dominant inheritance ● Congenital molecular genetic defect involving specific ion pumps or chloride channels (Clcn7) in the plasma membrane of osteoclasts ● Defect causes abnormal breakdown of bone tissue ● Resultant excessive new bone formation ● Diminished elasticity of bone.
Two types of manifestation and four subtypes:
Osteopetrosis with precocious manifestations.
– Infantile (malignant) form (autosomal recessive).
– Delayed osteopetrosis.
Albers–Schönberg disease (autosomal dominant).
– Intermediate recessive form.
– Intermediate recessive form, combined with renal tubular acidosis and mental retardation.

Imaging Signs

▶ **Modality of choice**
Radiography.

▶ **Pathognomonic findings**
Marked diffuse osteosclerosis.

▶ **Radiographic findings**
Abnormally high bone density ● Generalized density and thickening of the entire skeletal system except the mandible ● Diminished difference in transparency between the medullary space and cortex ● Club-like expansion of the metaphyses of long tubular bones ● Lucent bands may be found in metaphyseal regions ● There may be a "bone-within-bone" appearance ● Sclerotic bands along inferior and superior vertebral end plates ("sandwich vertebral body" appearance) ● Thickened and strongly sclerotic calvarial bones and skull base ● Noticeable difference between sclerotic maxilla and normal density of mandible ● Premature ossification of hyoid bone ● Absent or diminished pneumatization of the paranasal sinuses and mastoid.

▶ **MRI findings**
Not relevant ● May be an incidental finding ● Bone is hypointense on both T1-weighted and T2-weighted sequences due to marked sclerosis.

▶ **Nuclear medicine**
Nonspecific accumulation of ^{99m}Tc-phosphonate in skull base, long bones (humerus, femur, tibia), shoulder, and pelvis.

Fig. 5.16 Adult form of osteopetrosis in a 36-year-old male. Lateral thoracic radiograph. Incidental finding. Sclerotic bands along the vertebral end plates as well as central circumscribed sclerosis producing a "bone-within-bone" appearance in the vertebral body. Note also the sclerosis of the ribs.

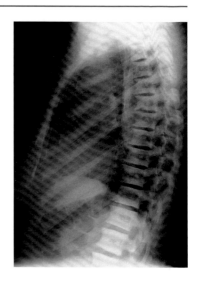

Clinical Aspects

▶ **Typical presentation**

Symptoms vary according to type ● Anemia ● Susceptibility to infection ● Reactive hepatosplenomegaly (extramedullary hematopoiesis) ● Cranial nerve pareses (narrowing of skull base foramina) ● Albers–Schönberg disease often asymptomatic ● Tendency to fracture (poor bone quality) ● Increased incidence of osteomyelitis.

▶ **Treatment options**

Allogenic stem cell transplantation (osteoclasts develop from hematopoietic stem cells in the bone marrow) ● Symptomatic: low-calcium and low-vitamin-D diet (in infants, discontinue vitamin D prophylaxis immediately).

▶ **Course and prognosis**

Infantile (malignant) form: neonatal manifestation ● Seizures ● Blindness and deafness in the first year of life are possible initial presenting signs ● Dramatically reduced life expectancy without treatment ● Survival rate to age 6 is 30% ● Most common causes of death are hemorrhage and infection, owing to insufficient hematopoiesis.

Other forms: Late onset of symptoms or incidental finding ● Manifestation usually at puberty ● Slightly decreased life expectancy.

▶ **What does the clinician want to know?**

Extent of involvement ● Fractures ● Rule out osteoblastic metastasis.

Differential Diagnosis

Osteomyelofibrosis	– Difficult to distinguish; sclerosis is usually more inhomogeneous
Osteoblastic metastasis	– Patient history
	– No hepatosplenomegaly
	– Usually includes destructive osseous changes
	– Sclerosis is more inhomogeneous
Mastocytosis	– Patient history (flushing attacks)
	– No splenomegaly
	– Radiographs: diffuse/focal sclerosis or diffuse/focal osteopenia

Tips and Pitfalls

Misdiagnosing as osteoblastic metastasis or osteomyelofibrosis, which can sometimes be difficult to distinguish.

Selected References

Vanhoenacker FM, De Beuckeleer LH, Van Hul W, et al. Sclerosing bone dysplasias: genetic and radioclinical features [review]. Eur Radiol 2000; 10(9):1423–1433

Kornak U, Mundlos S. Genetic disorders of the skeleton: a developmental approach [review]. Am J Hum Genet 2003; 73(3): 447–474

Definition

▶ **Epidemiology**
Synonyms: juvenile kyphosis, adolescent kyphosis ● Incidence: 1–15% ● Manifestation usually at age 10–15 ● Boys more often affected than girls.

▶ **Etiology, pathophysiology, pathogenesis**
Poor quality of cartilaginous ring apophysis of the vertebral end plate, predominantly affecting the thoracic vertebrae and thoracolumbar spine ● Intervertebral disk herniations into the vertebral body at areas of weakness in the cartilaginous ring apophysis (Schmorl nodule and vertebral body depression, usually anterior, leading to wedge vertebrae).

Imaging Signs

▶ **Modality of choice**
Radiography.

▶ **Pathognomonic findings**
Increased thoracic kyphosis with irregular, undulating vertebral body end plates and Schmorl nodules.

▶ **Radiographic findings**
Increased thoracic kyphosis ● Undulating irregularies on vertebral body end plates, mainly on anterior aspects ● Schmorl nodes at center of vertebral body or along anterior margin (retromarginal prolapse) ● Possible increased bone growth on the contralateral end plate (Edgren–Vaino sign) ● Sometimes increased longitudinal vertebral body diameter ● Decreased anterior disk space height.

▶ **MRI findings**
Vertebral body end plate collapse or detection of Schmorl nodes with presence of disk material within vertebral body ● In acute herniation, adjacent marrow edema (hyperintense on fat-saturated images and hypointense on T1-weighted images) ● Degeneration of the intervertebral disk: dehydration, hence hypointense on T2-weighted images.

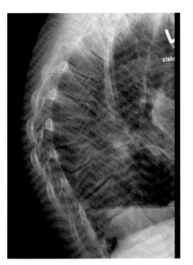

Fig. 5.17 Adolescent kyphosis (Scheuermann disease). Lateral radiograph of the spine in a 14-year-old boy. Typical irregularities on the anterior aspects of the inferior and superior vertebral body end plates of the mid-thoracic spine as well as small Schmorl nodes. The kyphosis of the thoracic spine curve measures 69°.

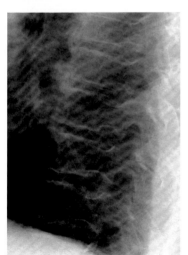

Fig. 5.18 Abnormal involution of the notochord. Lateral radiograph of the spine (detailed view). The depressions on the vertebral end plates are located posteriorly and in contrast to Scheuermann disease have shallow undulations.

Developmental Disorders

Clinical Aspects

▶ **Typical presentation**
   Thoracolumbar/lumbar involvement often painful even in early-stage disease ●
   Forms with thoracic involvement often painless ● Kyphosis.
▶ **Treatment options**
   Rigid kyphosis less than 50° may be treated with postural exercises and/or physical therapy ● Brace therapy for kyphotic curvature of 50–80° ● Operative treat-
   ment may be required for severe kyphotic angulation (> 80°).
▶ **Course and prognosis**
   Rigid thoracic kyphosis under 50°: unproblematic, possible esthetic concerns
   (especially women) ● Thoracic kyphosis greater than 50°: back pain possible,
   especially in the lumbar region, resulting from biomechanical disturbances
   (compensatory hyperlordosis) ● Kyphotic angulation greater than 70° can progress even in adulthood.
▶ **What does the clinician want to know?**
   Kyphotic angle: angle between superior vertebral end plate of T3 and inferior
   vertebral end plate of T11 ● Normal: 20–40°.

Differential Diagnosis

Abnormal involution of notochord	– Vertebral end plate defects on posterior aspects of the vertebral bodies
	– Depressions form shallower undulating appearance
Eosinophilic granuloma, tumors	– Changes limited to one vertebral body
	– No disk narrowing
	– Osteolytic lesions
	– On MRI, signal alterations typical of tumor
Osteochondrosis	– No undulating irregularities on vertebral end plates
	– Spondylosis
	– Narrowing of disk space

Tips and Pitfalls

Misdiagnosis as tumor in patients with recent vertebral body collapse or osteochondrosis.

Selected References

Blumenthal SL, Roach J, Herring JA. Lumbar Scheuermann's. A clinical series and classifi-
   cation. Spine 1987; 12(9): 929–932
Lowe TG. Scheuermann's disease [review]. Orthop Clin North Am 1999; 30(3): 475–487, ix
Wenger DR, Frick SL. Scheuermann kyphosis [review]. Spine 1999; 24(24): 2630–2639

Definition

▶ **Epidemiology**
Usually manifests during early childhood • Incidence is 10.8 per 100 000 among white children aged 0–15 years • Incidence among black children is 0.45 per 100 000 • Boys are affected four times as often as girls • Peak incidence: age 4–8.

▶ **Etiology, pathophysiology, pathogenesis**
Etiology is not entirely understood • Genetic factors play a role • Other suggested factors include increased intra-articular and intraosseous pressure, coagulation disorders, and immunoglobulins • Primary disorder: aseptic necrosis of the femoral head, decreased height, and fragmentation, possibly trauma-related (circumflex femoral artery).

Imaging Signs

▶ **Modality of choice**
Radiographs (AP and axial images).

▶ **Radiographic findings**
Changes not radiographically detectable until a minimum of 4 weeks after symptom onset • Classification by purely morphological radiographic features.
Classification by course:
– Condensation stage: femoral head is more radiodense and flattened than normal • Widened joint space (effusion, associated synovitis) • Lateralization of the femoral head • Delayed ossification of epiphyseal nucleus • Soft-tissue swelling.
– Fragmentation stage: deterioration and fragmentation of the femoral head • Zones of osteolysis and sclerosis • Flattening and widening of the femoral head • Metaphyseal cysts.
– Repair stage: repair of the femoral head.
– Final stage: with or without defect healing • Spherical, cylindrical, or mushroom-shaped femoral head • Shortened femoral neck • Proximalized greater trochanter.
Caterall classification system based on extent of femoral head involvement:
– Stage I: anterolateral quadrant (good prognosis).
– Stage II: anterior one-third to one-half.
– Stage III: up to three-quarters, posterior remains intact (worst prognosis due to very marked flattening).
– Stage IV: entire femoral head.
Signs of potential collapse of the epiphysis ("head-at-risk" signs):
– Gage's sign: V-shaped zone of osteopenia on the lateral epiphysis.
– Lateral calcifications.
– Horizontal epiphyseal plate.
– Lateralization of femoral head.

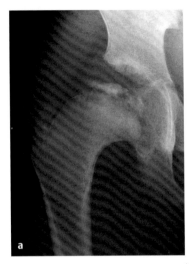 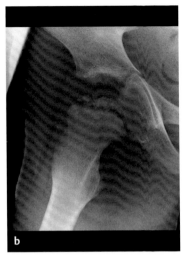

Fig. 6.1 a, b Perthes disease affecting the right side. Fragmentation stage. **a** AP and **b** axial radiographs of right hip joint. Moderate centering of slightly lateralized femoral head. Joint effusion. Metaphyseal lucency and incipient lateral calcifications ("head-at-risk" sign).

Stulberg classification system of increasing osteoarthritis risk related to increasing femoral head deformity and hip joint incongruity:
– Stage I: round femoral head • Normal size.
– Stage II: round femoral head • Coxa magna.
– Stage III: oval/mushroom-shaped femoral head • Coxa magna.
– Stage IV: flattened femoral head • Congruence of hip joint preserved.
– Stage V: flattened femoral head • Incongruence of hip joint.

▶ **MRI findings**
If clinical suspicion is present despite uncertain radiographic findings • In early stages, epiphysis displays diffuse signal decrease on T1-weighted sequences • Irregular signal intensity especially in subchondral areas • Cartilage thickening may be seen • As disease progresses, reconversion of fatty marrow signal • Effusion • Synovitis • Good visualization of extent of necrosis and slight femoral head deformities.

▶ **Nuclear medicine**
Decreased accumulation with impaired blood supply to femoral head • Increased activity during repair stage.

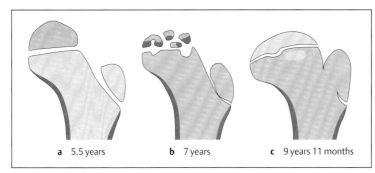

Fig. 6.2 a–c Stages in Perthes disease.
a Condensation stage.
b Fragmentation stage, followed by repair with consolidation and disappearance of fragmentation.
c Final stage.

Clinical Aspects

▶ **Typical presentation**
Limping and mild to moderate hip pain • Acute (in 25% after trauma) or persisting for several weeks • Adduction and flexion position • Usually marked restriction of range of motion in the affected hip, mainly reduced abduction and internal rotation.

▶ **Treatment options**
Treatment measures have three objectives:
  – Improve range of motion: physical therapy • Mobilization under anesthesia • Hydraulic mobilization • Adductor lengthening • Extension with increasing abduction.
  – Relieve weight bearing (controversial).
  – Centering methods (improve hip joint congruity, "containment"): abduction orthoses (controversial) • Intertrochanteric osteotomy • Pelvic osteotomy.

▶ **Course and prognosis**
Outcome varies considerably, ranging from spontaneous revascularization with full recovery to coxa plana and fragmentation of the femoral head with formation of secondary degenerative changes and loose intra-articular bodies • Follow-up is necessary regardless of treatment method • Clinical check-ups every 3 months • Radiographic follow-up (AP and axial views) every 6 months until 2 years after diagnosis, then annually • AP radiograph again at skeletal maturity • Most significant prognostic factors are age (good prognosis if onset before age 6), subluxation, lateral calcification, mobility (worse prognosis with severely limited range of motion), sex (delayed results worse in girls than boys) • In up to 20% bilateral, usually not symmetrical.

▶ **What does the clinician want to know?**
Diagnosis ● Disease stage ● Treatment progress.

Differential Diagnosis

(Spondylo-)epiphyseal dysplasia	– Bilateral, symmetrical deformities – Usually manifests in second year of life
Hypothyroidism	– Bilateral, symmetrical deformities
Osteochondritis dissecans	– Rarely involves hip – Usually affects older children – Usually small, well-marginated fragment
Coxitis	– Marked effusion – Clinical findings – MRI: marked edema and soft-tissue reaction

Tips and Pitfalls

Failing to recognize the "head-at-risk" sign.

Selected References

Moens P, Fabry G. Legg-Calvé-Perthes disease: one century later. Acta Orthop Belg 2003; 69(2): 97–103

Pillai A, Atiya S, Costigan PS. The incidence of Perthes' disease in Southwest Scotland. J Bone Joint Surg Br 2005; 87(11): 1531–1535

Scherl SA. Common lower extremity problems in children. Pediatr Rev 2004; 25(2): 52–62

Definition

Synonym: spontaneous aseptic osteonecrosis of the knee

▶ **Epidemiology**
Disease affecting older patients (6th and 7th decades) ● Women affected three times as often as men ● Unilateral in 99%.

▶ **Etiology, pathophysiology, pathogenesis**
Aseptic osteonecrosis of the weight-bearing portion of the medial femoral condyle ● Less often (< 15%) affects the lateral femoral condyle or medial tibial plateau ● Etiology unclear ● Possibly due to disrupted blood supply, repetitive microtrauma, or stress fracture.

Imaging Signs

▶ **Modality of choice**
Conventional radiography ● MRI.

▶ **Radiographic findings**
Initial flattening of the condyle or epiphysis ● In later stages, subchondral, usually crescent-shaped, lucency with reactive sclerosis ● Subchondral bone plate usually preserved.

▶ **MRI findings**
In early disease, signs of edema followed by demarcation ● Areas of necrosis are hypointense on all sequences ● Smaller lesion size (< 4 × 14 mm) generally related to good prognosis ● In later stages, flattened femoral condyle.

Clinical Aspects

▶ **Typical presentation**
Acute onset, severe pain without remembered trauma, especially at night and when resting ● Usually unilateral ● Pain limits range of motion.

▶ **Treatment options**
Valgus-producing osteotomy and core decompression ● Endoprosthesis if appropriate.

▶ **Course and prognosis**
Prognosis worsens with increasing size of affected area ● Good prognosis for lesions up to 3.5 cm^2 ● Worse prognosis in lesions larger than 5 cm^2 or if more than 50% of the medial condyle surface is involved ● Complications: articular surface collapse, genu varum, and secondary gonarthrosis.

▶ **What does the clinician want to know?**
Size of necrotic lesion ● Collapse ● Secondary degenerative changes.

Fig. 6.3 a–d
Osteonecrosis of
the knee in a 65-
year-old woman.
Sudden onset of
severe pain without
trauma.
a AP and **b** lateral
radiographs of the
knee showing radio-
lucent area (arrow)
with surrounding
sclerosis, degenera-
tive changes, and
vaguely flattened
articular surface.

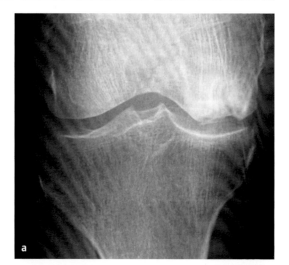

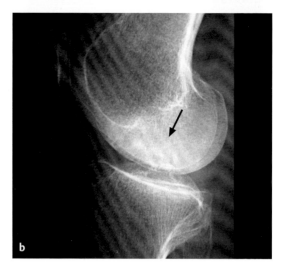

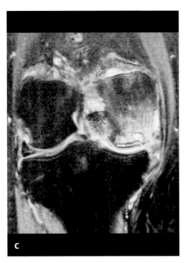
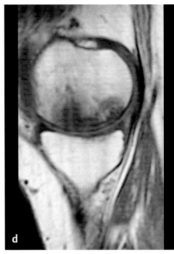

c,d MRI. Coronal fat-saturated proton density-weighted (**c**) and sagittal T1-weighted (**d**) images. Perifocal edema and linear subchondral area indicating a (stress) fracture along with degenerative changes in the medial meniscus.

Differential Diagnosis

Osteochondritis dissecans	– Affects adolescents – Usually toward the medial aspect of the condyles (intercondylar groove)
Transient bone marrow edema syndrome	– No demarcation – Migration possible in course of disease
Subchondral stress fracture	– Linear hypointense band (all sequences) parallel to subchondral bone plate

Tips and Pitfalls

False-negative diagnosis in early disease; mistaking disease for osteochondritis dissecans.

Selected References

Aglietti P, Insall J, Bohne WH. Idiopathic osteonecrosis of the knee: aetiology, prognosis and treatment. J Bone Joint Surg Br 1983; 65: 588–597

Lecouvet FE, Malghem J, Maldague BE, Vande Berg BC. MR imaging of epiphyseal lesions of the knee: current concepts, challenges and controversies. Radiol Clin North Am 2005; 43(4): 655–672

Narváez JA, Narváez J, De Lama E, Sánchez A. Spontaneous osteonecrosis of the knee associated with tibial plateau and femoral condyle insufficiency stress fracture. Eur Radiol 2003; 13: 1843–1848

Pape D, Seil R, Kohn D, Schneider G. Imaging of early stages of osteonecrosis of the knee. Orthop Clin North Am 2004; 35(3): 293–303

Watson RM, Roach NA, Dalinka MK. Avascular necrosis and bone marrow edema syndrome [review]. Radiol Clin North Am 2004; 42(1): 207–219

Definition

▶ **Epidemiology**
Peak incidence at age 20–40 ● Men affected twice as often as women ● Incidence: 1 in 100 000.

▶ **Etiology, pathophysiology, pathogenesis**
Avascular osteonecrosis ● Chronic repetitive microtrauma (e.g., working with a jackhammer) ● Idiopathic ● After a single traumatic event ● Constitutional ulna minus variant (variance > 2 mm, 50% of patients) ● Marked bone remodeling ● Coexisting areas of osteoclastic resorption and osteoblastic bone formation ● Between these are usually well-circumscribed areas of bone necrosis and cysts (zones of necrotic debris) on proximal lunate ● Growth of fibrovascular tissue into damaged area ● Fibrocartilage along the marginal zones represents an attempt by the body to counteract complete devitalization.

Imaging Signs

▶ **Modality of choice**
Radiographs of the wrist in two planes ● MRI.

▶ **Radiographic findings**
Findings often unremarkable in early stages.
Decoulx staging:
  – Stage 0: no radiological changes.
  – Stage I: increased radiodensity with preservation of bone contours.
  – Stage II: cancellous bone sclerosis and development of pseudocysts.
  – Stage III: fragmentation of proximal lunate.
  – Stage IV: progressive sintering and perilunate necrosis.

▶ **MRI findings**
For early recognition of the osteonecrosis.
  – Stage I (Stage 0 in radiography): marrow edema (hypointense on T1-weighted images, hyperintense on T2-weighted and fat-saturated sequences) ● Enhancement after contrast administration is a sign of vitality ● Potentially reversible.
  – Stage II: partial necrosis (patchy areas of enhancement after contrast administration).
  – Stage III: complete necrosis (hypointense on T1-weighted, T2-weighted SE and GE images, no enhancement after contrast administration) ● Sintering.

Fig. 6.4 Slight ulna minus variance in a 28-year-old man with a 1-year history of pain and swelling about the wrist joint. AP wrist radiograph demonstrating sclerosis and fracture of the lunate. Stage III lunatomalacia.

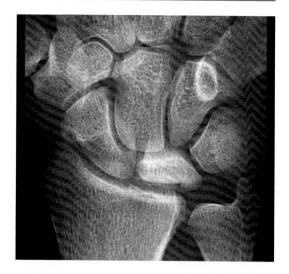

Fig. 6.5 Stage I lunatomalacia in a 38-year-old man. MRI, T1-weighted SE image. Hypointense signal intensity is consistent with bone marrow edema.

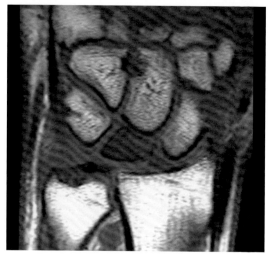

Clinical Aspects

▶ **Typical presentation**
Pain on weight bearing ● Limited range of motion ● Swelling ● Diminished strength ● Pain due to axial compression of the continuation of the third digital ray.

▶ **Treatment options**
In patients with ulna minus variance, radial shortening osteotomy (decompression and improvement of lunate vascularization) ● In early disease (stages 0–I) decompression and immobilization ● Lunate resection and capitate distraction ● Lunate resection and replacement with coiled tendon or Swanson Silastic implant as placeholder ● Arthrodesis in advanced osteoarthritis.

▶ **Course and prognosis**
Complications: severe wrist arthritis ● Pain, even on resting, that is not responsive to treatment ● Permanent limitation of wrist motion.

▶ **What does the clinician want to know?**
Stage ● Ulna minus variant ● Signs of arthritis.

Differential Diagnosis

Lunate fracture	– Clearly related to trauma
	– Sharp radiolucent line
	– No areas of dense bone sclerosis
Secondary lunate ossification center	– Rounded, smooth border
	– No areas of dense bone sclerosis

Selected References

Bonzar M, Firrell JC, Hainer M, Mah ET, McCabe SJ. Kienböck disease and negative ulnar variance. J Bone Joint Surg Am 1998; 80(8): 1154–1157

Zanetti M, Saupe N, Nagy L. Role of MR imaging in chronic wrist pain. Eur Radiol 2007; 17(4): 927–938

Definition

Synonyms: avascular, ischemic, aseptic femoral head necrosis in the adult
- **Epidemiology**

  Manifests between ages 25–55 • Peak incidence: age 35 • Affects men four times as often as women • Incidence in Europe: 0.01% • In up to 70% of cases, metachronic involvement of contralateral hip.
- **Etiology, pathophysiology, pathogenesis**

  Multifactorial etiology arising from diminished vascular supply to the femoral head (medial femoral circumflex artery), predisposing underlying disease, risk factors, and mechanical stresses • Ultimately vascular insufficiency of the subchondral region • Abnormal permeability • Vascular stasis • Bone marrow edema • Increased intraosseous pressure.
  - Post-traumatic femoral head necrosis (vessel rupture after femoral neck fracture, hip dislocation).
  - Non-traumatic femoral head necrosis (fat or air emboli, increased intramedullary pressure).

  Predisposing underlying diseases (20–50%): decompression sickness • Sickle-cell anemia • Gaucher disease • Radiation therapy • Systemic lupus erythematosus • Steroid therapy • Cushing disease.

  Risk factors (50–80%): pancreatitis • Alcohol abuse • Pregnancy • Hypofibrinolysis • Hypercoagulability • Abnormal lipid metabolism.

Imaging Signs

- **Modality of choice**

  MRI: early diagnosis and in stages 0–II (sensitivity is 89%, specificity is 100%) • Coronal slices of both hip joints to exclude involvement of contralateral hip • High resolution • Two planes • Affected hip joint including sagittal sections for treatment planning (position, size of lesion).

  Radiography: stage III and later.
- **Radiographic findings**

  ARCO (Association Research Circulation Osseous) classification (histology; radiographs, CT, or MRI with reference to size and location; nuclear medicine).
  - Position: A = medial, B = central, C = lateral.
  - Involvement of femoral head circumference: A < 15%, B = 15–30%, C > 30%.
  - Extent of femoral head collapse or flattening: A < 2 mm, B 2–4 mm, C > 4 mm.

  Stage 0 (initial stage): Histologic evidence of osteonecrosis • No changes in morphologic appearance.

  Stage I (early, reversible stage): Radiography and CT: normal appearance • Nuclear medicine: diffuse tracer uptake or "cold spots" • MRI: bone marrow edema without demarcation around avascular zone.

  Stage II (early, irreversible stage): Radiography and CT: sclerotic margin, focal sclerosis, asterisk sign • Nuclear medicine: "cold-in-hot" spot • MRI: demarcation of reactive peripheral zone with "double line" sign (in 65–80%): T2-weighted images show a linear zone of high signal intensity toward the marginated lesion (vascularized granulation tissue) and one of low signal intensity toward surrounding bone (sclerosis); on noncontrast T1-weighted sequences, both are hypointense and there is enhancement of the vascularized zone after contrast administration.

Stage III (transitional stage): Radiography (e.g., Lauenstein view) and CT: subchondral radiolucent line (crescent sign), flattening of femoral head, subchondral fracture • Nuclear medicine: "hot-in-hot" spot • MRI: flattening of femoral head, linear, high (fluid-filled fracture gap) or low (dense trabeculae) signal intensity under the subchondral bone plate (crescent sign: subchondral fracture).

Stage IV (late stage): Radiography, CT, and MRI: collapse of articular surfaces, secondary degenerative changes • Nuclear medicine: hot spot.

Clinical Aspects

▶ **Typical presentation**
Symptoms range in severity from "numbness" of the hip to persistent pain with inability to walk • Gradual onset of resting pain, increasing under mechanical stress • Joint effusion • After articular surface collapse, alternating episodes of acute and mild pain.

▶ **Treatment options**
  – Stages 0–II: Relieve weight bearing • Possible anticoagulation therapy • Core decompression.
  – Stages II–IV: Core decompression • Corrective osteotomy • Bone transplantation • Vascularized graft • Joint replacement.

▶ **Course and prognosis**
Arthritis related to site affected (main weight-bearing zone) and local extent (> 30% of articular surface) • Femoral head infarction leads to irreversible damage • If untreated: in more than 85% of cases, progression within 2 years; in more than 50%, articular surface collapse and secondary arthritis.

▶ **What does the clinician want to know?**
Diagnosis • Size and position of articular surface involvement.

Fig. 6.6a–d
Femoral head ne-
crosis in ARCO stage
III C disease affect-
ing more than 30%
of the surface of
the femoral head.
The lesion is located
(anterosupero-)
laterally.

a, b Pelvic radio-
graph (**a**) and axial
projection of the hip
joint (**b**) showing
secondary degener-
ative changes. In **b**
there is a faint sub-
chondral radiolu-
cent line in the cen-
tral femoral head
circumference.

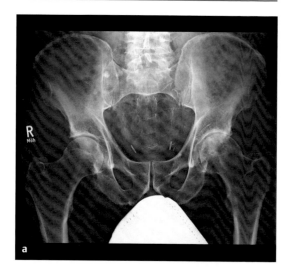

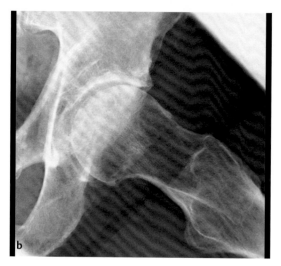

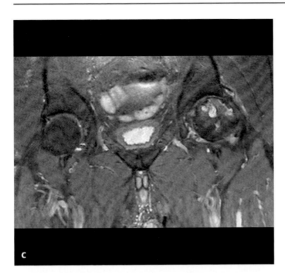

c,d MRI. Coronal STIR (**c**) and coronal T1-weighted (**d**) images. Wedge-shaped area with a sclerotic margin which is hypointense on T1-weighted images (**d**) and hyperintense in parts on STIR images (**c**). Incipient flattening of the femoral head.

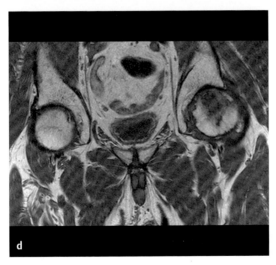

Differential Diagnosis

Perthe disease	– Ischemic osteonecrosis of femoral head epiphysis
	– Predilection for boys aged 4–8 years
Transient osteoporosis (bone marrow edema syndrome)	– Sudden onset of hip pain
	– Self-limiting in 9–12 months
	– Diffuse marrow edema
	– Often marked involvement of femoral neck
	– No demarcation in course of disease
Stress fracture	– Patient history (unusual mechanical stress or osteopenia)
	– Fracture line, typical localization (inferomedial femoral neck cortex)
Osteomyelitis	– Increased inflammatory parameters
	– Extensive soft-tissue involvement
	– Erosive changes

Tips and Pitfalls

Delayed diagnosis owing to initially unremarkable radiographic findings, and thus delayed initiation of treatment.

Selected References

Assouline-Dayan Y, Chang C, Greenspan A, Shoenfeld Y, Gershwin ME. Pathogenesis and natural history of osteonecrosis. Semin Arthritis Rheum 2002; 32(2): 94–124

Ficat RP. Idiopathic bone necrosis of the femoral head; early diagnosis and treatment. J Bone Joint Surg Br 1985; 67B(1): 3–9

Mankin HJ. Nontraumatic necrosis of bone (osteonecrosis) [Current Concepts review]. N Engl J Med 1992; 326(22): 1473–1479

Mont MA, Hungerford DS. Non-traumatic avascular necrosis of the femoral head [Current Concepts review]. J Bone Joint Surg Am 1995; 77(3): 459–474

Watson RM, Roach NA, Dalinka MK. Avascular necrosis and bone marrow edema syndrome. Radiol Clin North Am 2004; 42(1): 207–219

Definition

▶ **Epidemiology**
Affects men twice as often as women ● Bilateral involvement in 30% of cases.

▶ **Etiology, pathophysiology, pathogenesis**
Demarcation and possible detachment of an osteochondral fragment, usually along the concave side of articular bones ● Complete detachment results in a free intra-articular osteochondral fragment known as a "joint mouse."

– Juvenile form: more common ● Rarely before age 10 ● Epiphyseal plates still open.
– Adult form: less common ● After reaching skeletal maturity.
– Systemic form: multiple lesions on several joints.
– Common sites: distal femur ● Trochlea of talus ● Radial head.

Etiology unclear ● Possibly due to repetitive microtrauma and/or vascular factors (end arteries) ● Hormonal and genetic factors under discussion ● High potential for repair in younger patients.

Imaging Signs

▶ **Modality of choice**
Radiographs (AP and lateral; for knee involvement also tunnel view to visualize the intercondylar fossa) ● MRI to assess fragment stability.

▶ **Radiographic findings**
Findings depend on stage of disease ● Radiographic staging follows Berndt and Harty, using the ankle joint as an example:

– Stage I: unremarkable.
– Stage II: well-demarcated, crescent-shaped or oval area of increased radiolucency surrounded by a sclerotic margin and mostly firmly anchored to the bone.
– Stage III: detached, undisplaced fragment.
– Stage IV: loose intra-articular fragment ("joint mouse"), lesion bed is empty.

▶ **MRI findings**

– Stage I: edema.
– Stage II: demarcation of subchondral area.
– Stage III: partial detachment of osteochondral fragment.
– Stage IV: complete detachment of osteochondral fragment, nondisplaced.
– Stage V: displacement of osteochondral fragment from lesion bed.

Stages I and II are stable ● Stages IV and V are unstable ● Stability of stage III lesions is difficult to assess, but clinically relevant.

– Sign of stability: linear zone of hyperintense signal corresponding to area of enhancement after contrast administration (granulation repair tissue between fragment and crater).
– Signs of instability: linear signal zone that is isointense to fluid on T2-weighted images, larger than 5 mm, and continuous (via cartilage and subchondral bone) with the joint space ● Subchondral cysts larger than 5 mm ● Chondromalacia.

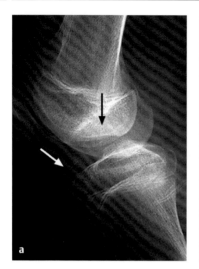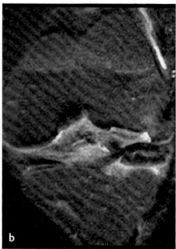

Fig. 6.7 a, b Osteochondritis dissecans in a 5-year-old boy.
a Lateral radiograph of the knee joint. Large osteochondral fragment (white arrow) with corresponding defect on the femoral condyle (black arrow).
b MRI, coronal STIR image. The displaced fragment has become attached to the anterior horn of the lateral meniscus.

Clinical Aspects

▶ **Typical presentation**
Nonspecific symptoms ● Pain usually related to weight bearing ● Limited range of motion ● Joint stiffness ● Intra-articular loose bodies may cause locking.

▶ **Treatment options**
Apart from patient age (potential for repair) and lesion size and location (weight-bearing zone), fragment stability is the determining factor in the choice of treatment ● Underlying principles of treatment include avoidance of weight bearing, revitalization of the lesional area, reattachment of the fragment, and implantation of replacement tissue.
Conservative: Relieve weight bearing, e.g., with crutches ● Physical therapy ● Good healing potential in juvenile form.
Surgical: Drilling ● Subchondral spongiosaplasty ● Fragment reattachment (resorbable pins, fibrin glue) ● Osteosynthesis with metal implants (possibly spongiosaplasty) ● OATS plasty.

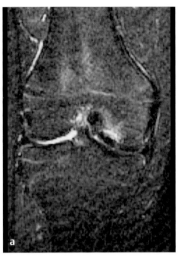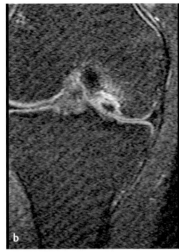

Fig. 6.8 a, b   Osteochondritis dissecans. MRI.
a Coronal STIR sequence showing a linear zone of signal intensity that is isointense to fluid. The space between the lesion and surrounding bone exceeds 5 mm, but there is no continuity with the joint cavity. Small cartilage defect.
b Postcontrast coronal fat-saturated T1-weighted image. Enhancement between the bone and the defect, consistent with granulation tissue and thus representing active repair.

▶ **Course and prognosis**
  Prognosis depends on disease stage and patient age ● More favorable prognosis in younger patients with small, stable lesions not involving main weight-bearing zones ● Prearthritic deformity not always avoidable ● Spontaneous remission is possible.

▶ **What does the clinician want to know?**
  Location ● Size ● Stability.

Osteonecrosis

Differential Diagnosis

Osteonecrosis	– No detached fragment
	– Topography of lesions
Transient bone marrow edema syndrome	– No demarcation
	– Migration possible during course of disease
Subchondral stress fracture	– Linear hypointense band (all sequences) parallel to subchondral bone plate
Chondromatosis	– Typical cartilaginous, possibly punctate calcified matrix
	– Rounded appearance of chondromas

Tips and Pitfalls

Mistaking disease for an ossification disorder, especially in younger children.

Selected References

Kutcha-Lissberg F, Singer P, Vescei V, Marlovits S. Osteochondritis dissecans of the knee joint. Radiologe 2004; 44(8): 783–788

Santrock RD, Buchanan MM, Lee TH, Berlet GC. Osteochondral lesions of the talus. Foot Ankle Clin 2003; 8(1): 73–90

Wall E, Von Stein D. Juvenile osteochondritis dissecans. Orthop Clin North Am 2003; 34(3): 341–353

Definition

▶ **Epidemiology**

Ischemic necrosis ● Usually an incidental finding diagnosed after the 4th decade ● Most commonly affects long-bone metaphyses (usually femur, tibia, or humerus) ● May extend far into the diaphysis (up to 20 cm in length) ● Purely epiphyseal bone infarct is rare ● Typically symmetrical involvement.

▶ **Etiology, pathophysiology, pathogenesis**

Impaired blood supply to the bone (intraluminal obstruction, vessel compression or rupture) ● Vascular occlusion ● Polycythemia vera (increased blood viscosity) ● Hemoglobinopathies ● Hypocorticalism ● Pancreatitis ● Exposure to extreme cold ● Severe burn trauma ● Radiation therapy ● Decompression sickness (nitrogen emboli).

Imaging Signs

▶ **Modality of choice**

Radiography ● MRI.

▶ **Radiographic findings**

In early stages, osteopenia and loss of cancellous bone with surrounding sclerotic rim ● Patchy sclerosis arising from sintering of necrotic bone and reactive new bone formation ● In later stages, irregular, patchy opacities or calcifications (pebble, cluster-of-grapes, chain-like, or ring-like appearance), usually located peripherally ● Infarction may measure up to 20 cm in length ● In epiphyseal infarction, tongue-like or wedge-shaped opacities extending from their bases on articular surfaces ● Possible collapse of articular surfaces.

▶ **CT findings**

Trabecular destruction ● Usually an incidental finding.

▶ **Nuclear medicine**

In early disease, decreased accumulation at necrotic site ("cold spot") ● Later, also increased uptake ("cold-in-hot" spot).

▶ **MRI findings**

In early stages, edema (hypointense on T1-weighted images and hyperintense on T2-weighted images) ● Later, demarcation along the periphery (hypointense on T1-weighted images; on T2-weighted images hyperintense line toward necrosis, corresponding to granulation tissue) ● Hypointense line toward healthy bone (sclerosis, fibrosis): "double-line" sign ● Enhancing peripheral zone ● In older bone infarcts, the signal intensity of the necrotic zone is equal to that of fat ● Peripheral zone typically serpiginous, resembling a garland.

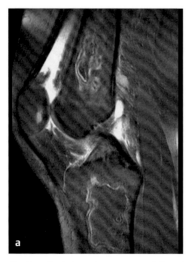 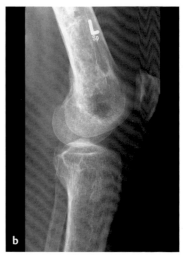

Fig. 6.9 a, b Mature bone marrow infarction.

a Sagittal fat-saturated proton density-weighted MRI. The image shows a garland-like sclerotic margin and a central area of fatty marrow signal. The multiple necrotic zones are mainly located in the metadiaphyseal region, but there are also a few directly below the joint, hence there is a risk of articular surface collapse.

b Radiograph showing faint sclerotic margin and central area of decreased radiodensity in the distal femur and in the tibia. The proximal femur demonstrates areas of somewhat coarse sclerosis which are occasionally difficult to differentiate from enchondroma.

Clinical Aspects

▶ **Typical presentation**
  Usually asymptomatic ● Rarely, uncharacteristic localized pain.

▶ **Treatment options**
  Usually does not require treatment ● In subarticular infarction with joint surface collapse, reconstruction of the articular surface may be carried out.

▶ **Course and prognosis**
  Very rarely, development of sarcoma after bone infarction.

▶ **What does the clinician want to know?**
  Location ● Size ● Rule out differential diagnoses.

Differential Diagnosis

Enchondroma	– Lobulated, cluster-of-grapes appearance – Fine, dotted, or comma-shaped areas (calcifications) of decreased signal intensity scattered over central portions of the lesions
Chondrosarcoma	– Highly differentiated forms resemble enchondroma, biopsy if diagnosis uncertain
Infection (early stage)	– No periosteal reaction – Signal intensity resembling that of edema on MRI – Even recent infarction often well-circumscribed without surrounding reaction

Tips and Pitfalls

Mistaking bone infarct for one of the differential diagnoses requiring treatment.

Selected References

Lafforgue P, Schiano A, Acquaviva PC. Bone infarction, or idiopathic metaphyseal and diaphyseal aseptic osteonecrosis of the long bones. Update and contribution of new imaging technics [in French]. Rev Rhum Mal Osteoartic 1990; 57(4):359–366

Pere P, Regent D, Vivard T, Gillet P, Gaucher A. Magnetic resonance imaging of bone infarction. Apropos of 2 cases [in French]. J Radiol 1988; 69(10): 597–601

Saini A, Saifuddin A. MRI of osteonecrosis. Clin Radiol 2004; 59(12): 1079–1093

Definition

▶ **Epidemiology**
Incidence of traumatic meniscal lesions is 61 in 100 000 ● 60% of people over age 60 have degenerative meniscal lesions ● 80% of meniscal lesions involve the medial meniscus ● Predilection for posterior regions ● Combined medial and lateral tears are rare (< 10%) ● Frequently combined with lesions involving the anterior cruciate ligament (35–78%) ● Longitudinal tears are more common than transverse tears.

▶ **Etiology, pathophysiology, pathogenesis**
Traumatic or degenerative ● Predisposition in professions involving kneeling (e.g., tilers) and professional athletes ● Rupture occurs when applied force (peak force) cannot be absorbed by internal joint structures ● Often involve rotational movement with slight flexion of the knee joint ● Depending on the severity of trauma, may be combined with cruciate ligament rupture, collateral ligament rupture, or osteochondral fractures.

Classification based on morphological criteria:

– Types of tears: longitudinal, transverse, radial, lobulated, bucket-handle (extensive longitudinal tear in which the detached fragment remains fixed to the anterior and posterior horns, but is displaced within the intercondylar space), complex tear.

– Location: anterior, middle, or posterior third of the circumference, medial or peripheral third.

Imaging Signs

▶ **Modality of choice**
MRI ● Sensitivity and specificity about 90% ● Diagnosis and preoperative planning (location, type, extent).

▶ **Radiographic findings**
Radiography to exclude bone involvement ● At most, secondary degenerative changes.

▶ **MRI findings**
SE or TSE sequences with short echo time ● GE sequences often false-positive ● Often associated with cartilage lesions and signal alterations resembling bone marrow edema.

Classification of signal abnormalities (usually increased signal) by their appearance:

– Grade 0: normal findings.

– Grade I: foci of increased signal not extending to the surface.

– Grade II: linear zone of increased signal intensity that does not extend to the surface.

– Grade III: focal or linear zone of increased signal intensity that reaches the meniscal surface.

– Grade IV: several areas of increased signal intensity that reach the surface; fragmented meniscus.

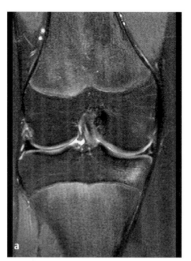 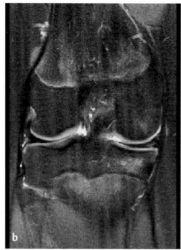

Fig. 7.1 a, b Post-traumatic meniscal tear. Fat-saturated TSE proton density-weighted MRI. **a** Intermediate coronal and **b** posterior coronal images. Extensive rupture (longitudinal components measuring more than 15 mm) in intermediate portion and posterior horn of the medial meniscus. The extent of the lesion and presence of additional transverse components (**b**) (complex tear) are suggestive of instability.

Diagnosis of a tear in grade III or IV lesions is most accurate when changes are depicted in more than one slice and more than one plane.

Signs of instability: extent greater than 1 cm (one-third of meniscal circumference) • Fragment displacement • Complex tear (multiplanar).

Clinical Aspects

▶ **Typical presentation**

Pain on extension • Favoring the affected joint in a flexed position • Limited function (weight bearing, mobility, locking) • Effusion • Swelling • Hemarthrosis.

Clinical tests: pain provocation on compression of joint space (Böhler sign, Payr sign, Steinmann II sign: posterior horn) or the application of shear forces (Steinmann I sign).

▶ **Treatment options**

Conservative treatment for small, basically asymptomatic stable lesions • Operative treatment consists of meniscal suture (peripheral third) or resection of lesions with irreparable mobile fragments, preserving as much of the meniscus as possible.

▶ **Course and prognosis**

If left untreated, mechanically relevant lesions are associated with increased risk of secondary arthritis since menisci absorb up to 40% of the load transmitted from the femur to the tibia.

Fig. 7.2 a–e Meniscal tear patterns.
a Longitudinal.
b Vertical, beginning at the apex and curving radially toward the base.
c Transverse with fish-mouth tear.
d Bucket-handle tear.
e Complex tear with radial and longitudinal components as well as fragment displacement.

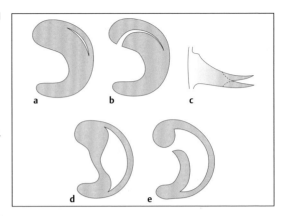

Fig. 7.3 Classification of signal alterations seen in meniscal lesions.

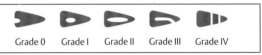

Grade 0   Grade I   Grade II   Grade III   Grade IV

▶ **What does the clinician want to know?**
Diagnosis • Type of lesion and severity • Additional bony or cartilaginous changes.

Differential Diagnosis

MRI generally enables precise differentiation of meniscal lesions from other disorders (e.g., gonarthrosis, knee ligament injuries, osteochondritis dissecans, rheumatoid arthritis, gout, fractures, intra-articular loose bodies, and synovitis).

Tips and Pitfalls

False-positive diagnosis on MRI due to transverse ligament, section through popliteal tendon or meniscofemoral ligament, or uncertainty about whether signal alterations reach the surface • False-negative findings in post-traumatic slight radial tears of the posterior horn of the lateral meniscus.

Selected References

Bin SI, Kim JM, Shin SJ. Radial tears of the posterior horn of the medial meniscus. Arthroscopy 2004; 20(4): 373–378

Cothran RL Jr, Major NM, Helms CA, Higgins LD. MR imaging of meniscal contusion in the knee. AJR Am J Roentgenol 2001; 177(5): 1189–1192

Forster MC, Aster AS. Arthroscopic meniscal repair. Surgeon 2003; 1(6): 323–327

Fritz RC. MR imaging of meniscal and cruciate ligament injuries. Magn Reson Imaging Clin N Am 2003; 11(2): 283–293

Harper KW, Helms CA, Lambert HS 3rd, Higgins LD. Radial meniscal tears: significance, incidence, and MR appearance. AJR Am J Roentgenol 2005; 185(6): 1429–1434

Definition

▶ **Epidemiology**
Anterior cruciate ligament usually affected in knee injuries • Rupture of thicker posterior cruciate ligament less common • In 70% the tear is in the middle portion of the cruciate ligament • Incidence in Germany is 32 per 100 000 • Usually affects younger people and athletes (e.g., soccer or football, skiing) • NB: in more than 50% of cases combined with meniscal, collateral ligament, and/or osteochondral injury.

▶ **Etiology, pathophysiology, pathogenesis**
Twisting trauma (rotation of the tibia against the femur) in flexion • Hyperextension injuries may also damage posterior cruciate ligament, and possibly posterolateral joint capsule structures (e.g., popliteal tendon, lateral collateral ligament, or biceps tendon) • Failure of ligamentous structures occurs when acute peak force exceeds mechanical stability and elongation reserve • Passive subluxation and impaction of the femur and tibia against each other • Resulting excessive translation ("drawer") of tibia against femur • Contusion sites depend on mechanism of injury.

Imaging Signs

▶ **Modality of choice**
Radiographs in two planes • Tunnel view may be useful to clarify bony lesions after knee trauma • MRI.

▶ **Radiographic findings**
Avulsion fracture of anterior or posterior cruciate ligament from the tibial attachment only • Typically seen in children • May be recognized by a fragment that is often minimally displaced upward into the intercondylar groove (if the fragment is hidden by bone a careful search must be made) • Impaction fracture (> 2 mm) on lateral femoral condyle (middle third: "deep notch" sign) is specific for anterior cruciate ligament rupture.

▶ **MRI findings**
Views in all three main imaging planes • Paracoronal plane sometimes also useful.
Direct signs of rupture: High sensitivity • Disrupted continuity • Wavy contour • Abnormal course • Ill-defined • Edematous • Absent from normal anatomic position.
Indirect signs of rupture: High sensitivity • Excessive curvature and increased angulation of posterior cruciate ligament (sagittal images generally demonstrate concave superior margin of posterior cruciate ligament; normal ligament has elongated convex superior margin) • Anterior translation of tibia against femur exceeding 7 mm • Posterior subluxation of posterior horn of lateral meniscus beyond the posterior margin of the tibial cortex • Contusions (even osteochondral fracture) on posterolateral tibial plateau and possibly also intermediate portion of lateral femoral condyle; in extreme trauma, corresponding findings also in medial compartment • In posterior cruciate ligament rupture, contusions on anterior aspect of tibia and anterior part of femoral condyle.

Fig. 7.4 a–d   Anterior cruciate ligament rupture.
a Sagittal, **b** paracoronal, and **c** axial MRI images. Thickened ligament with discontinuity in proximal third (**a, b**). Contusions on posterolateral tibial plateau and slight contusions also on the lateral femoral condyle (**a**) with a small impression fracture on the posterior end of the lateral tibial plateau (**c**).

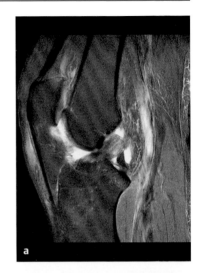

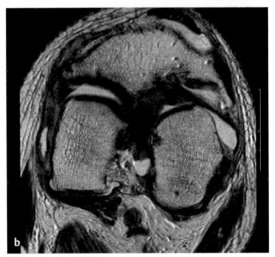

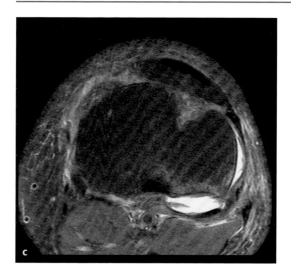

Clinical Aspects

▶ **Typical presentation**
Pain ● Knee swelling ● Hematoma ● Instability ("giving way") ● Anterior translation ● Positive Lachman test.

▶ **Treatment options**
Conservative: passive physical therapy ● Orthopedic devices.
Surgical: cruciate ligament reconstruction (arthroscopic or open) with semitendinosus (pure tendinoplasty) or patellar tendon (bone–tendon–bone graft) ● Screw fixation for bony avulsion.

▶ **Course and prognosis**
Good prognosis given successful reconstruction and muscular compensation ● High risk of arthritis in patients with persistent instability ● Satisfaction largely depends on level of athletic activity: 75% of patients who are not very physically active are satisfied without reconstruction surgery while the same is true for only 15% of highly active patients.

▶ **What does the clinician want to know?**
Diagnosis of cruciate ligament rupture ● Additional injuries (menisci, osteochondral lesions, additional ligamentous lesions that imply instability) ● Bony avulsion.

Intra-articular Lesions

Fig. 7.5 Radiograph showing bony avulsion of the tibial attachment of the anterior cruciate ligament in a child. A careful search must be made for such injuries since the bone fragment may be hidden in the intercondylar groove.

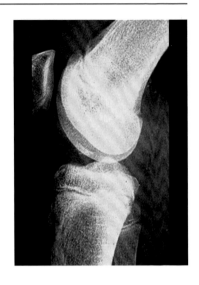

Differential Diagnosis

In general, MRI (with radiography as the basic examination) enables precise diagnosis of acute intra-articular knee injury.

Tips and Pitfalls

Mistaking fat deposits at the tibial attachment site of the anterior cruciate ligament for (partial) rupture • Missing a bony avulsion injury • Missing combined injuries (especially meniscal lesions).

Selected References

Fritz RC. MR Imaging of meniscal and cruciate ligament injuries. Magn Reson Imaging Clin N Am 2003; 11(2): 283–293

Moore SL. Imaging of the anterior cruciate ligament. Orthop Clin North Am 2000; 33(4): 663–674

White LM, Miniaci A. Cruciate and posterolateral corner injuries in the athlete: clinical and magnetic resonance imaging features. Semin Misculoskelet Radiol 2004; 8(1): 111–131

Definition

▶ **Epidemiology**
Post-traumatic and in asymptomatic athletes in 20–50% of arthroscopically examined patients ● Detected on MRI studies in up to 80% of patients with osteoarthritis.

▶ **Etiology, pathophysiology, pathogenesis**
Causes of cartilage damage include:
- Acute trauma leading to direct cartilage injury and sometimes subchondral bone.
- Repeated physical stress (wear and tear).
- Enzymatic factors.

Cartilage is bradytrophic tissue with only a very limited potential for repair ● Quality and quantity of biosynthesis (chondrocytes) is controlled by enzymatic and biomechanical (deformation) factors ● A cartilage lesion usually leads to a process of progressive cartilage degeneration ● Cartilage defects disrupt the congruity of the joint surface and thus constitute a prearthritic deformity.

Imaging Signs

▶ **Modality of choice**
MRI ● Direct MR arthrography ● Direct CT arthrography.

▶ **MRI findings**
The most comprehensive sequences for evaluating cartilage are moderate fat-saturated T2-weighted TSE sequences and fat-saturated T1-weighted or water-excitation (WE) 3D GE sequences:
- Moderately fat-saturated T2-weighted sequences profit from the high signal intensity of joint fluid, which forms a contour around the cartilage ("arthrographic effect") and highlights any irregularities on the cartilage surface.
- T1-weighted FS/WE 3D GE sequences profit from high spatial resolution, which at 1.5 T can be up to $1.5 \times 0.3 \times 0.3 \, mm^3$; they are very good at distinguishing cartilage from subchondral bone.

Imaging subchondral areas with signal intensity resembling that of bone marrow edema is helpful when searching for neighboring cartilage lesions.

Findings depend on the stage of cartilage damage ● In the mildest injuries, only intracartilaginous signal alterations are present ● Focal cartilage swelling with intact surface ● Fissuring ● Mild surface irregularities ● Gradual reductions in thickness (foci representing defects, or diffuse thinning) are given in intervals of half of the absolute cartilage thickness ● In final stages, exposure and erosion of subchondral bone ● In addition to lesional depth, surface area and compartmental involvement are also included.

▶ **Direct CT arthrography findings**
Joint distention allows better depiction of discontinuity. In joints with a thin layer of cartilage (e.g., hip joint, elbow, and ankle) the higher spatial resolution of CT is advantageous.

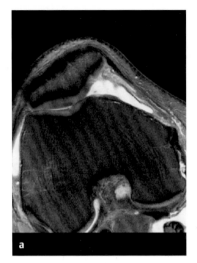

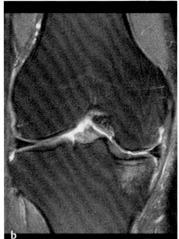

Fig. 7.6 a–c Various grades of cartilage damage. Fat-saturated T2-weighted MRI.
a Post-traumatic chondral lesion with focal edematous fibrillation.
b Moderate loss of cartilage substance.
c Loss of cartilage down to the subchondral bone accompanied by subchondral edema.

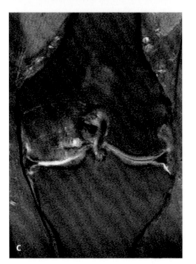

Clinical Aspects

▶ **Typical presentation**

Related to traumatic or degenerative joint damage • No correlation between cartilage damage and amount of pain • There may be initiation or exacerbation of degenerative changes as a result of cartilage damage • Loose bodies (cartilage flakes) may cause locking or catching and are usually found in the joint capsule recess.

▶ **Treatment options**

Lavage • Debridement • Microfracture • AOT (autologous osteochondral transplantation) • ACT (autologous chondrocyte transplantation) • Corrective osteotomy • Partial or complete endoprosthesis • Macroscopically intact cartilage, small fissures, and minimal articular surface depressions are managed conservatively • Osteochondral fractures with notable step-offs on the articular surface and larger detached fragments/defects require surgical treatment.

▶ **Course and prognosis**

Criteria for appropriate treatment and prognosis:

– Location, size of area involved, severity and number of chondral defects (grading).
– Associated meniscus, bone, and ligament injuries as well as axis deviations.
– Age and patient's desired level of physical activity.

▶ **What does the clinician want to know?**

Grading • Overall status of affected joint.

Tips and Pitfalls

Over- or underestimating cartilage damage.

Selected References

Fritz RC. MR Imaging of meniscal and cruciate ligament injuries. Magn Reson Imaging Clin N Am 2003; 11 (2): 283–293

Moore SL. Imaging of the anterior cruciate ligament. Orthop Clin North Am 2000; 33(4): 663–674

White LM, Miniaci A. Cruciate and posterolateral corner injuries in the athlete: clinical and magnetic resonance imaging features. Semin Musculoskelet Radiol 2004; 8(1): 111–131

Definition

▶ **Epidemiology**
Incidence of shoulder dislocation (most common cause of labral lesions): 1–2% of the population ● About two-thirds of lesions involve the anteroinferior quadrant (Bankart lesion, anterior labroligamentous periosteal sleeve avulsion [ALPSA], glenolabral articular disruption [GLAD]) ● Incidence of superior labrum anterior to posterior (SLAP) lesions is 3–10%.

▶ **Etiology, pathophysiology, pathogenesis**
Labrum and capsule provide stability to the shoulder joint ● Labrum augments the glenoid cavity to help receive the humeral head ● Labral lesions are generally caused by trauma, usually acute and severe, less often repetitive trauma (e.g., throwing sports).

Shoulder dislocation: Anteroinferior shoulder dislocation usually followed by lesion in anteroinferior quadrant (Bankart, ALPSA, Perthes lesion) ● Incidence is 10 in 100 000 ● Often with impaction fracture of posterosuperior humeral circumference (Hill–Sachs lesion).

Bankart lesion: Avulsion of the labrum with or without bony component from the glenoid cavity ● Bankart lesions, anterior labral periosteal sleeve avulsion (ALPSA), and Perthes lesions vary in terms of extent of injury of inferior glenohumeral ligament and periosteum.

GLAD lesion: Caused by forced adduction with externally rotated, abducted arm ● Anteroinferior labral rupture with adjacent cartilage injury.

SLAP lesion: Caused by sudden traumatic arm abduction or repeated overhead arm movements (posterosuperior impingement) ● Commonly seen in tennis, volleyball, and baseball players ● Typical trauma: fall onto outstretched arm with slightly abducted and flexed shoulder.

- SLAP I: Degenerative labral fraying ● Limited at attachment of biceps tendon ● 10% ● Questionable clinical relevance ● Uncertain differentiation from sublabral recess.
- SLAP II: Tear extends anteriorly or posteriorly beyond the attachment of the biceps tendon ● Parallel to glenoid circumference ● Up to the level of the medial glenohumeral ligament ● Unstable biceps anchor ● 40%.
- SLAP III: Intra-articular displacement of detached labrum ● Comparable to bucket-handle tear ● Site of attachment of biceps tendon intact ● 30%.
- SLAP IV: Similar to SLAP III with additional rupture of the long biceps tendon ● Displacement of the tendon or a portion of it into the joint space ● 15%.
- SLAP V: Longitudinal tear beginning superiorly and extending anteriorly and far inferiorly.
- SLAP VI: Longitudinal tear with loose end of the labrum hanging in the joint space ("flap tear").
- SLAP VII: Longitudinal tear extending anteriorly and into the medial glenohumeral ligament.

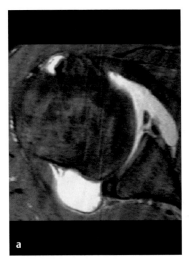 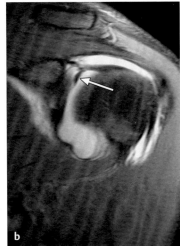

Fig. 7.7 a, b   Axial fat-saturated proton density-weighted MRI. Anteroinferior labral lesion with periosteal stripping. Slightly thickened posterior labrum with central degeneration (**a**). Coronal fat-saturated proton-density-weighted MRI. SLAP III lesion with a fragment (arrow) hanging in the joint space similar to a bucket-handle lesion (**b**).

Imaging Signs

▶ **Modality of choice**
Conventional radiography as basic diagnostic procedure ● In acute injuries, unenhanced MRI with joint effusion serving as a "natural contrast agent" ● Otherwise direct MR arthrography ● Alternatively, direct CT arthrography.

▶ **Radiographic findings**
Possible to visualize dislocation and bone injuries as well as reduction result ● Bony Bankart lesion with fragment in sublabral recess ● Hill–Sachs lesion on posterosuperior humeral head ● Direct imaging of position of a dislocated humerus (inferior, anterior, and medial) ● Posteriorly dislocated humerus will show the trough line sign (vertical oblique radiodense line in the humeral head), absence of the half-moon overlap between humeral head and glenoid, and may show a "reverse" Hill–Sachs lesion with anterosuperior impaction fracture of the humeral head.

▶ **MRI findings**
Examination or reconstruction in all three planes is essential ● Careful alignment of the imaging plane with the level of the labral opening facilitates assessment ● Linearly increased signal intensity with interrupted labral contour ● A bone fragment may be detected ● Rolled-up portions of damaged capsule, ligaments, or periosteum may be seen.

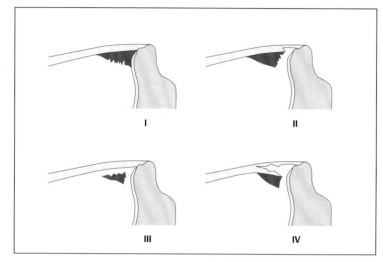

Fig. 7.8 Classification of labral lesions (coronal plane). SLAP I and II: lesion without displacement. SLAP III and IV: migration of fragment into joint space without (III) or with portions of the biceps tendon (IV).

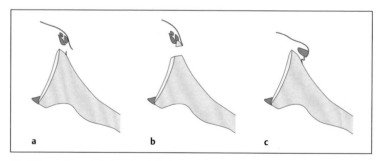

Fig. 7.9 a–c Anteroinferior glenoid lesions.
a Complete separation of capsule and labrum from the glenoid cavity.
b Additional separation of a portion of bone from the glenoid cavity.
c Intact capsule and periosteal components lead to inferomedial displacement of torn labrum.

▶ **CT arthrography findings**
Findings correspond to MRI ● Lesions are hyperdense relative to surrounding structures.

Clinical Aspects

▶ **Typical presentation**
Shoulder symptoms may be nonspecific ● Pain ● Cracking or snapping sounds with motion ● Predominant feature is instability.

▶ **Treatment options**
Arthroscopic smoothing and debridement ● Suturing or reattachment of detached labrum ● In SLAP lesions, possible repair of biceps anchor ● Screw fixation of bony Bankart lesion ● Capsule tightening for atraumatic instability.

▶ **Course and prognosis**
Good prognosis if treated early.

▶ **What does the clinician want to know?**
Diagnosis ● Distinguish from normal anatomical variants ● Location and extent ● Precise differential diagnosis of various types of lesions is often difficult—the most important task is to clarify the presence and location of the lesion.

Differential Diagnosis

Sublabral foramen	– Well-circumscribed labral detachment of variable size along the anterosuperior glenoid cavity from 1 to 4 o'clock
	– Usually follows the contour of the glenoid cavity
	– Extends vertically or somewhat proximally
	– Limited to anterosuperior two-thirds of the labrum
Buford complex	– Partial labral aplasia with thickened medial glenohumeral ligament
	– Misinterpretation can be avoided by systematically imaging all structures from craniad to caudad
Sublabral recess	– Observed in 80% of shoulders
	– Uncertain differentiation from SLAP I
	– Typically, smooth rim around the labrum
Wide joint capsule	– Overdistended capsule illustrating the redundancy of capsular structures as cause of atraumatic instability (usually only recognized on direct arthrography)

Tips and Pitfalls

Mistaking the intermediate signal of the labral base, produced by the hyaline carti-lage extending to it, for labral detachment ● Mistaking a sublabral recess, a subla-bral foramen, or Buford complex for a SLAP lesion ● False-negative diagnosis with unenhanced MRI studies.

Selected References

Jbara M, Chen Q, Marten P, Morcos M, Beltran J. Shoulder MR arthrography: how, why, when [review]. Radiol Clin North Am 2005; 43(4):683–692, viii

Pfirrmann C. MRT der Schulter [in German]. Radiologie Up2date 2001; 1: 125–143

Snyder SJ, Karzel RP, Del Pizzo W, Ferkel RD, Friedman MJ. SLAP lesions of the shoulder. Arthroscopy 1990; 6(4): 274–279

Definition

▶ **Epidemiology**
Collective term describing lesions ranging from small degenerative changes to extensive ruptures with secondary retraction and atrophy • Rupture frequency after trauma: 5% in patients under age 50 and up to 80% in those over age 80 • In older individuals, trauma such as (sub-)luxation tends to lead to rotator cuff rupture while in younger people labral lesions are more common • Usually involves the supraspinatus tendon, much less commonly the tendons of the subscapularis (usually trauma-related) or infraspinatus.

▶ **Etiology, pathophysiology, pathogenesis**
Tears may be classified as follows:
  – Complete tear: full-thickness tear that connects the joint cavity with the subacromial space, irrespective of affected size of area.
  – Partial tear: articular, on the bursal side, or interstitial.
Extensive tears may lead to fatty atrophy and/or degeneration as well as retraction of affected muscles.
Degenerative tear: Most common type • Risk factors are age, (sub-)acromial anatomy, impingement, and pre-existing rotator cuff lesions • Lesions affecting the distal supraspinatus tendon may lead to diminished blood supply • Arm position and activity in certain professions may play a role.
Traumatic tear: Less common • Shoulder dislocation or sudden abduction of the arm against resistance.

Imaging Signs

▶ **Modality of choice**
MRI • MR arthrography.

▶ **Radiographic findings**
High-riding humeral head (acromiohumeral distance < 6 mm) may be seen in full-thickness rotator cuff tears • Erosions on inferior surface of acromion from high-riding humeral head • Flattening and atrophy of greater tubercle due to absent tensile forces.

▶ **MRI findings**
High diagnostic certainty in full-thickness rotator cuff tears • Sensitivity: 75–100% • Very reliable assessment of lesion size • Unenhanced MRI studies are less reliable in distinguishing partial tears or small full-thickness tears from tendinopathy (MR arthrography is superior).
Demonstration of defect contours with hyperintense fluid signal on fat-saturated T2-weighted and STIR sequences • There may be leakage of fluid or contrast medium through the defect into the subacromial and/or subdeltoid bursa • Where lesions are small, degeneration may lead to overestimation of the extent of the lesion • Sequences with short echo times may lead to overestimation of the extent of the lesion due to minimal contrast between the tear (fluid) and degeneration as well as the "magic angle" effect.

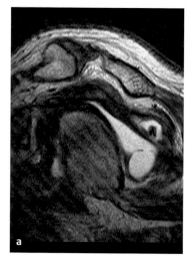

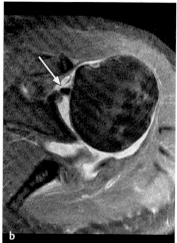

Fig. 7.10 a–c Advanced rotator cuff destruction with underlying degenerative changes. Torn supraspinatus and subscapularis tendons, medially displaced long biceps tendon, and marked atrophy of all muscles contributing to the rotator cuff.
a Sagittal MRI. Generalized atrophy, caudally displaced belly of the subscapularis, and displacement of the biceps tendon into the joint.
b Axial MRI. Displaced biceps tendon and "empty sulcus" appearance (arrow).
c Coronal MRI. Portions of the ruptured supraspinatus tendon "floating" just superolateral to the biceps tendon.

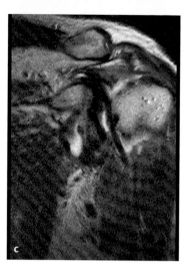

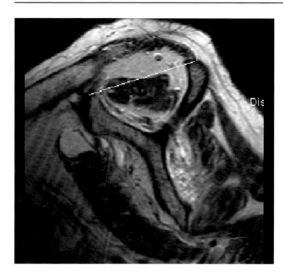

Fig. 7.11 Defect arthropathy in torn rotator cuff. Sagittal MRI. Advanced glenohumeral arthritis. Marked atrophy of the supraspinatus muscle and borderline positive "tangent sign," i.e., the tangent to the coracoid process and the spina scapulae does not cross the supraspinatus muscle belly.

Degenerative changes without rupture: Ill-defined area of increased signal • There may be thickening of the affected portion of the tendon without disrupted contour or presence of signal intensity isointense to fluid • Typical location is 1 cm from the attachment of the supraspinatus muscle—exactly where the tendon passes obliquely to the main magnetic field • MRI scan protocols should thus include a sequence with a long echo time which diminishes artificially increased signal resulting from the "magic angle" effect.

Rupture: Tear extending in two planes • Tendon and muscle retraction • Precise descriptions should be given of any muscle exhibiting fatty degeneration or atrophy (on T1-weighted images: replacement of muscle tissue by hyperintense fat signal, decreased muscle belly diameter) • Lesions typically begin at the anterior supraspinatus tendon and extend posteriorly into the infraspinatus tendon or anteroinferiorly into the superior margin of the subscapularis tendon • In traumatic subscapular tendon tears, consider possible displacement of the biceps tendon (usually deep and medial, and less often superficial, to the subscapular tendon).

Intra-articular Lesions

Clinical Aspects

▶ **Typical presentation**
  Shoulder pain • Restricted shoulder abduction.

▶ **Treatment options**
  Choice of reconstructive method based on size of lesion • Smaller lesions may be treated with arthroscopy, other lesions with open reconstruction • If symptom relief takes precedence over restoration of function, conservative therapy (physical therapy) or arthroscopic debridement may be considered.

▶ **Course and prognosis**
  Prognosis after reconstructive surgery depends on muscle condition (atrophy and/or fatty degeneration) • Poor prognosis associated with fatty atrophy and degeneration of more than 50% of the transverse diameter of a muscle; retraction of tendon ends to the level of the glenoid; older ruptures larger than 5 cm ("massive rupture"); or a high-riding humeral head with an acromiohumeral distance of less than 6 mm.

▶ **What does the clinician want to know?**
  Extent (complete or partial tear, length of defect) of lesion • Location of rupture • Affected tendons • Extent of muscle atrophy and tendon retraction • Quality of the tendon at the rupture site.

Differential Diagnosis

Calcific tendinitis	– Typical calcium deposit on radiographs
Subscapular nerve lesion	– Initial edema in infraspinatus muscle is consistent with denervation, then arthropathy and fatty degeneration
	– May be caused by ganglion

Tips and Pitfalls

Missing small full-thickness or partial tears, for which MRI diagnosis mainly relies on alterations in signal intensity (misinterpretation due to "magic angle" or partial volume effects) • Overestimating increased signal on T1-weighted sequences: presence of a lesion should not be assumed unless increased signal is also present on sequences with long echo times • Failing to describe a subscapularis lesion.

Selected References

Jbara M, Chen Q, Marten P, Morcos M, Beltran J. Shoulder MR arthrography: how, why, when [review]. Radiol Clin North Am 2005; 43(4): 683–92, viii

Kassarjian A, Bencardino JT, Palmer WE. MR imaging of the rotator cuff [review]. Radiol Clin North Am 2006; 44(4):503–23, vii-vii

Pfirrmann C. MRT der Schulter [in German]. Radiologie Up2date 2001; 1: 125–141

Definition

▶ **Epidemiology**
The lateral ligament is the most commonly injured ankle ligament, involved in 65–85% of ligamentous injuries • One of the commonest types of injury seen young athletes.

▶ **Etiology, pathophysiology, pathogenesis**
Partial or complete tear of the fibular capsule–ligament complex • May be followed by anterolateral ankle instability • Caused by supination trauma with plantar-flexed foot • Anterior talofibular and/or calcaneofibular ligament rupture first, less often the posterior talofibular ligament • Associated injuries: rupture of ankle joint capsule, osteochondral fractures of the talus, rupture of the anterior tibiofibular ligament (syndesmosis).

Imaging Signs

▶ **Modality of choice**
Radiographs of the ankle (lateral and AP views) • If fracture is ruled out, stress radiographs in two planes, comparing injured and uninjured sides • In exceptional circumstances, MRI and CT to detect associated injuries.

▶ **Radiographic findings**
Plain films: Evaluate for fractures and signs of degenerative joint changes • Rule out bony avulsion of the ligament (recent avulsion presents with osteopenia toward the tear margin, which has sharp corners) • Joint incongruity and/or joint space exceeding 6 mm indicate instability.
AP stress radiographs: Inversion stress • Angle between tibial plafond and talar trochlea is measured • Normal angle is less than 5°; 5–15° is uncertain; > 15° or a discrepancy greater than 8° between sides indicates ligamentous injury.
Lateral stress radiographs: Anterior talar translation • Shortest distance between posterior tibial lip and talar trochlea • More than 10 mm anterior translation or more than 5 mm difference between sides indicates ligamentous lesion.
Related findings: Osteochondral lesions on the talus often present as only faint osteopenia on the medial and lateral facets of the talar dome • In anterior impingement (delayed sequela), bone exostoses on the anterior tibial lip with reactive changes on the talar neck.

▶ **CT findings**
CT indicated mainly where there are associated bone injuries • Assessment of fragments • Intra-articular loose bodies.

▶ **MRI findings**
Good assessment of soft tissues • Complete rupture visible as disrupted and wavy-appearing ligament • Partial tears result in thickening and increased signal intensity • There may be an osteochondral lesion of the talus and (especially in severe trauma) a lesion opposite it on the distal tibia (hyperintense on T2-weighted images and hypointense on T1-weighted images; osteochondral fracture is a possibility) • Widened joint space and disruption of syndesmotic ligaments are signs of rupture • Effusion and soft-tissue swelling are usual • Direct

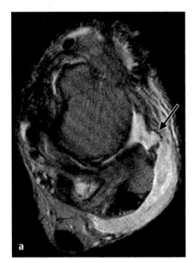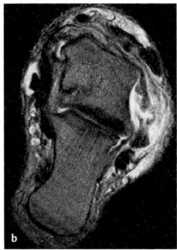

Fig. 8.1 a, b Lateral ankle ligament rupture. **a** Proximal and **b** distal paraxial MRI. Rupture of the anterior talofibular (**a**, arrow) and calcaneofibular ligaments (**b**), each showing disrupted and wavy appearance and lax portions. Joint effusion and soft-tissue swelling. Retinacular lesion (**b**).

MR arthrography will clarify presence of osteochondral lesions (cartilage covering, stability) and free cartilage or osteocartilage flakes ● Delayed sequelae: tarsal tunnel syndrome, anterior (bony) or anterolateral (soft-tissue) impingement.

Clinical Aspects

▶ **Typical presentation**
Pain ● Limited range of motion ● Instability ● Swelling.

▶ **Treatment options**
"Early functional" conservative treatment is the first-line choice: protective joint devices (brace, elastic bandage, orthosis) ● When appropriate, short-term plaster splint until swelling resolves ● Individualized weight-bearing exercises ● Physical therapy ● Coordination training ● Muscle strengthening ● NSAIDs to alleviate pain ● Primary surgery is uncommon; secondary surgery may be required in patients with chronic instability: fibular capsular ligament suture, primary ligament replacement surgery, or repair of fibular capsular ligaments.

▶ **Course and prognosis**
If untreated, lateral ligament rupture may lead to chronic instability with degenerative changes ● Impingement may occur.

▶ **What does the clinician want to know?**
Rule out fractures ● Bony avulsion of ligament ● Evaluation of talar tilt and anterior talar translation.

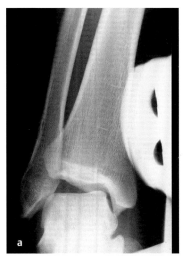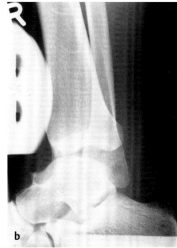

Fig. 8.2 a, b Stress radiographs in a patient with an ankle sprain: **a** AP and **b** lateral. Pathological joint laxity (**a**) and anterior talar translation (**b**) are signs of a ruptured anterior talofibular ligament and calcaneofibular ligament.

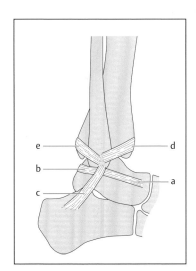

Fig. 8.3 a–e Anatomy of the lateral ligaments of the ankle.
a Anterior talofibular ligament.
b Posterior talofibular ligament.
c Calcaneofibular ligament.
Syndesmotic ligaments:
d Anterior tibiofibular ligament.
e Posterior tibiofibular ligament.

Differential Diagnosis

Ligament strain, fracture, chronic ligament instability, traumatic peroneal tendon dislocation, isolated syndesmotic rupture, Achilles tendon rupture.

Tips and Pitfalls

Misinterpreting an accessory ossicle as evidence of a bony avulsion.

Selected References

Becker HP, Rosenbaum D. Chronic recurrent ligament instability on the lateral ankle. Orthopäde 1999; 28(6): 483–492

Dunfee WR, Dalinka MK, Kneeland JB. Imaging of athletic injuries to the ankle and foot. Radiol Clin North Am 2002; 40(2): 289–312

Kirby AB, Beall DP, Murphy MP, Ly JQ, Fish JR. Magnetic resonance imaging findings of chronic lateral ankle instability. Curr Probl Diagn Radiol 2005; 34(5): 196–203

Definition

▶ **Epidemiology**
  Incidence is 20 in 100 000 • In Germany, about 16 000 cases per year • Age predilection: 30–50 years • Men are affected five times as often as women.

▶ **Etiology, pathophysiology, pathogenesis**
  Direct trauma, e.g., lateral blow to dorsiflexed foot • Laceration injury • Sudden
  impact • Indirect trauma (e.g., extreme muscle tension) with poor training technique or pre-existing degenerative changes (mainly in older athletes) • Increased risk after steroid injection or cytostatic use and in patients with connective tissue diseases, diabetes mellitus, chronic polyarthritis, and circulatory disorders.
  – Complete rupture • Most common form • Usually 2–6 cm above the calcaneal
    insertion site.
  – Partial rupture • Rare.
  – Avulsion fracture of the Achilles tendon from the calcaneus ("beak fracture") •
    Rare.

Imaging Signs

▶ **Modality of choice**
  Radiographs in two planes (rule out bony avulsion or other associated osseous
  injury) • Ultrasound • MRI.

▶ **Radiographic findings**
  Calcaneal fracture line if beak fracture is present • Soft-tissue swelling in the
  tendon (especially well seen on digital radiography: windowing!).

▶ **Ultrasound findings**
  Rupture appears as a gap in tendon • In partial ruptures, hematoma and inhomogeneous echo of the defect zone with a few remaining fibers.

▶ **MRI findings**
  Depiction of the entire Achilles tendon, especially if incomplete rupture suspected • Tendon thickening • Complete disruption • In later stages, areas of degeneration (tendinitis) and thinning • In incomplete rupture (rare), isolated, intra-
  tendinous partial fiber ruptures may be seen • Associated changes: bursitis, ten-
  donitis.

Clinical Aspects

▶ **Typical presentation**
  Whip-like, tearing pain when rupture occurs • Audible noise • Palpable gap over
  the tendon (depression) • Tenderness • Swelling • Hematoma • Unable to stand
  on toes • Loss of Achilles reflex.

▶ **Treatment options**
  Conservative: Increasingly common • Perhaps a cast for 1 week • Special shoe
  with anterior reinforcement and elevated heel (about 3 cm) for 6 weeks • Physical therapy with isometric strength training.

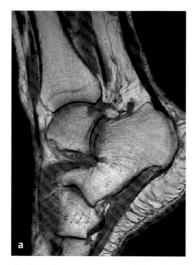 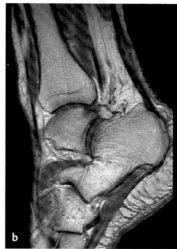

Fig. 8.4 a, b   Partial rupture of the Achilles tendon.
a T1-weighted MRI. Hyperintense spindle-shaped swelling in middle portion of the Achilles tendon.
b MRI after administration of contrast agent. The partial rupture is clearly demarcated by longitudinal and vertical areas of contrast enhancement.

Surgical: Especially in younger, active patients ● Suture ● Turndown flap ● Fibrin glue ● In beak fractures, reduction with screw fixation or tension-band wiring ● Short leg cast for 3–6 weeks after surgery.

▶ **Course and prognosis**
Return to sporting activities 3–4 months after conservative or operative therapy ● Competitive training after 6 months ● Risk of re-rupture is 2% after operative treatment ● Risk is up to 40% after conservative treatment.

▶ **What does the clinician want to know?**
Severity of rupture ● Skeletal involvement or other associated injuries.

Differential Diagnosis

Peritendinitis	– Fluid in surrounding soft tissues – Tendon is intact
Ankle fracture	– Visible fractures on radiography
Achilles bursitis	– Accumulation of fluid between Achilles tendon and calcaneus

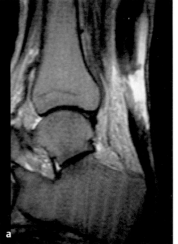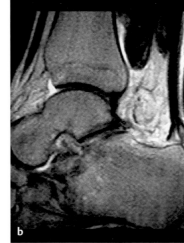

Fig. 8.5 a, b   MRI of a ruptured Achilles tendon.

a Complete rupture at the proximal end of the Achilles tendon near the myotendinous junction.

b Avulsion of the distal insertion of the tendon on the calcaneus.

Tips and Pitfalls

Missing associated bony injury or tendon dehiscence on post-treatment ultrasound follow-up.

Selected References

Järvinen TA, Kannus P, Paavola M, Järvinen TL, Jósza L, Järvinen M. Achilles tendon injuries. Curr Opin Rheumatol 2001; 13(2): 150–155

Karjalainen PT, Soila K, Aronen HJ, et al. MR imaging of overuse injuries of the Achilles tendon. AJR Am J Roentgenol 2000; 175: 251–260

Definition

▶ **Epidemiology**

Usually occurs in children and young athletes (age 12–16) ● Training error ● Affects nine times as many men as women (greater muscle mass).

▶ **Etiology, pathophysiology, pathogenesis**

Avulsion is a structural failure of the bone due to muscular pulling forces at a tendon attachment site or aponeurosis ● Apophysis is a "site of lessened resistance."

Acute avulsion fracture: Excessive, often eccentric muscle contraction ● Often related to intense recreational sports.

Chronic avulsion fracture: Repetitive microtrauma ● Overuse.

– Ischial tuberosity: origin of the hamstring muscles (biceps femoris, gracilis, semimembranosus, semitendinosus) ● Usually occurs before epiphyseal closure ● Forceful contraction (runners).

– Anterior superior iliac spine: attachment site of the sartorius and tensor fasciae latae ● Forceful extension of the hip joint (sprinters).

– Anterior inferior iliac spine: attachment site of the straight head of the rectus femoris ● Forceful extension of the knee joint (soccer players).

– Inferior pubic ramus: attachment of adductor longus, adductor brevis, and gracilis ● Usually chronic avulsion (soccer players).

– Intercondylar eminence: bony avulsion of cruciate ligament ● Children affected more often than adults ● Forced knee flexion with internal rotation.

– Tibial tuberosity: acute avulsion is uncommon ● Chronic avulsion: Osgood–Schlatter disease due to repeated microtrauma with traction of the patellar tendon on the tuberosity ● Athletically active adolescents (jumping, soccer) ● Bilateral in up to 50%.

– Inferior patellar pole: Sinding–Larsen–Johannson disease ● Pathogenesis similar to Osgood–Schlatter disease.

– Superior patellar pole: avulsion of quadriceps tendon ● Usually chronic avulsion injury in adolescents intensely active in sports.

– Medial humeral epicondyle: acute and chronic forms ● Sudden or repeated contraction of flexor-pronator muscle group ● Fall onto outstretched arm ● Affects adolescents.

– Base of fifth metatarsal bone: attachment of short peroneal tendon ● Forceful contraction with internally rotated foot.

– Segond fracture: cortical avulsion fracture on the lateral aspect of the tibial head ● Involvement of the meniscotibial portion of the lateral capsular ligament (middle third) ● Forceful internal rotation with varus stress.

Imaging Signs

▶ **Modality of choice**
Radiography usually sufficient when patient history and clinical presentation are typical ● Rotation and target radiographs often helpful ● MRI and bone scans are sensitive in early stages.

▶ **Radiographic findings**
Ischial tuberosity: curvilinear, sharply defined bone fragment ● In nondisplaced avulsion fractures, fragment is near original site (ischial epiphysiolysis) ● In displaced avulsion fractures, fragment displacement exceeds 2 cm ● During healing, "aggressive" appearance with areas of osteolysis and destruction.

- Inferior pubic ramus: usually chronic avulsions ● Prominent periosteal new bone formation ● No displaced fragments.
- Segond fracture: fragment usually visible on AP or tunnel views ● There may be a curved fragment (lateral capsule sign).
- Intercondylar eminence: often difficult to diagnose radiographically ● Supplementary tunnel and/or oblique views or CT/MRI.
- Medial humeral epicondyle: acute avulsion ● Soft-tissue swelling ● Displacement.
- Superior patellar pole: chronic avulsion ● Heterotropic ossification in the quadriceps tendon ● Fragmented superior border of the patella ● Soft-tissue swelling.
- Osgood–Schlatter disease: chronic avulsion ● Fragmentation of tibial tuberosity (distinguish from normal ossification center) ● Spiculation ● Soft-tissue swelling.

▶ **CT findings**
Helpful if radiographic findings are negative or injury is in subacute stage.

▶ **MRI findings**
Clarify associated injuries involving muscles, tendons, and ligaments ● Rule out malignancy where indeterminate osteolytic changes are shown.

- Pubis: usually unilateral findings (bone marrow edema) ● Soft-tissue proliferation on medial femur ● Strongly enhancing after administration of contrast material.
- Segond fracture: elliptical fragment below lateral tibial plateau ● Bone marrow edema along the medial tibial border ● Often combined with other significant knee injuries: anterior cruciate ligament rupture (75–100%), meniscal tear (66–70%), or fibular head avulsion.
- Osgood–Schlatter disease: soft-tissue swelling anterior to the tibial tuberosity ● Loss of sharp angle of infrapatellar fat body ● Thickening or edema affecting the inferior patellar tendon ● Infrapatellar bursitis.

Fig. 8.6 a, b
Avulsion fractures.
a Avulsion of the
rectus femoris from
the anterior inferior
iliac spine. Hetero-
tropic ossifications.
Displacement is less
than 2 cm.
b Avulsion of the
sartorius from the
anterior superior
iliac spine. Hetero-
tropic ossifications.
Displacement is less
than 2 cm.

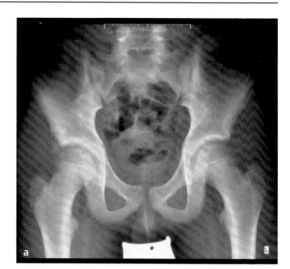

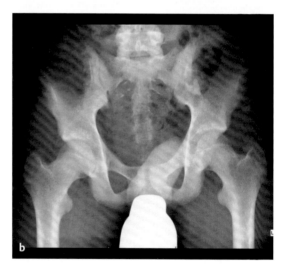

Clinical Aspects

▶ **Typical presentation**
Depending on affected site, pain may be related to weight-bearing ● In chronic forms, there may be diffuse, dull pain ● Night pain also possible.

▶ **Treatment options**
Immobilization of affected muscles ● Cooling ● Antiphlogistics ● Physical therapy with light stretching ● Surgery is usually not recommended.
– Ischial tuberosity: bed rest for several days ● Reduce activity ● Return to normal use in 6–12 weeks ● Poor prognosis in displaced avulsion injuries and when activity is not adequately reduced.
– Anterior superior/inferior iliac spine: good prognosis ● Temporarily reduced activity level (knee and hip flexion) ● Return to full use in 5–6 weeks.
– Medial humeral epicondyle: immobilization ● Fragment reduction ● Fragment realignment.

▶ **Course and prognosis**
Prognosis depends on adequate immobilization and avoidance of the triggering overuse or sport ● Displaced avulsion fractures of the ischial tuberosity carry the risk of fibrous bridging with restricted function ● There may be ischialgia arising from excessive callus formation or direct sciatic nerve impingement by the fragment.

▶ **What does the clinician want to know?**
Diagnosis ● Rule out tumor/inflammation (see differential diagnoses) ● Follow-up evaluation.

Differential Diagnosis

Osteomyelitis	– No association with typical overuse mechanisms
	– Patients usually adult
Bone tumor	– No association with typical overuse mechanisms
(e.g., Ewing sarcoma)	– Bone destruction

Tips and Pitfalls

Misinterpreting a healing avulsion fracture (with signs of periostitis) for osteomyelitis or a bone tumor. Even histologically, misdiagnosis as "well-differentiated osteosarcoma" is another potential pitfall. To avoid unnecessary biopsies, correct interpretation is vital. For this, clinical presentation and lesion topography are key ● Mistaking a displaced medial humeral epicondyle for an ossification center of the humeral trochlea.

Selected References

Donnelly LF, Bisset GS, Helms CA, Squire DL. Chronic avulsive injuries of childhood. Skeletal Radiol 1999; 28(3): 138–144

Stevens MA, El-Khoury GY, Kathol MH, Brandser EA, Chow S. Imaging features of avulsion injuries. Radiographics 1999; 19(3): 655–672

Definition

▶ **Epidemiology**
Pain in the shoulder joint on abduction and elevation due to mismatch between available space and path of motion • In 90% of cases subacromial • Supraspinatus tendon involved • Rarely subcoracoid.

▶ **Etiology, pathophysiology, pathogenesis**
Impingement of supraspinatus tendon between the roof of the subacromial space and the greater tubercle on abduction and elevation • Causes of subacromial narrowing include:
– Acromion shape.
– Subacromial osteophytes or osteophytes on the lateral clavicle (ACJ).
– Os acromiale.
– Bursitis, (peri-)tendinitis.
– High-riding humeral head.
– Diminished tendon perfusion.
– Prominent coracoid affecting the subscapularis muscle (coracoid impingement).
Acromion shape: Bigliani classification into three:
– Type I: flat.
– Type II: curved.
– Type III: hooked.
Types II and III are often associated with impingement • Acromion with gentle incline (< 75°) also associated with impingement.
Stages of impingement: Neer classification:
– Stage I: edema and hemorrhage in supraspinatus muscle (usually in patients under age 25).
– Stage II: tendinitis and fibrosis of rotator cuff • Thickening of subacromial bursa (patients aged 25–40 years).
– Stage III: rotator cuff tear (usually over age 40).

Imaging Signs

▶ **Modality of choice**
Radiographs • MRI.

▶ **Radiographic findings**
Views: AP, axial and outlet (to assess acromial shape), possibly Rockwood view • New bone formation • Osteophytes (spurs) on the undersurface of the acromion • Degenerative changes on the greater and lesser tubercles (flattening and sclerosis) • Calcifications at the attachment of the rotator cuff (calcific tendinitis) • Acromiohumeral distance may be diminished (normally > 10 mm) • Os acromiale may be present.

▶ **MRI findings**
Subacromial bursitis: acute effusion, double layer of fat in chronic bursitis • ACJ deterioration, especially capsular hypertrophy • Os acromiale • Shape of acromion • Depiction of bony changes along anterior margin of acromion and any

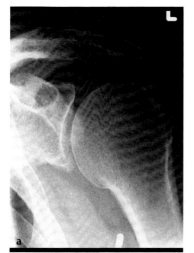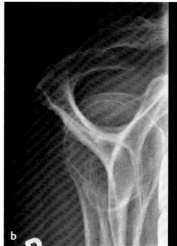

Fig. 8.7 a, b Shoulder impingement.

a Long-standing history of impingement. Subacromial osteophyte formation with mixed sclerotic/cystic appearance of the greater tubercle.

b Calcification at the origin of the coracoacromial ligament producing a sharp projection from the anterior end of the acromion.

associated changes of the rotator cuff • There may be signs of edema in patients with active arthritis affecting the ACJ.

Clinical Aspects

▶ **Typical presentation**
Diffuse shoulder pain and weakness, especially on abduction and external rotation • No history of trauma • Night pain • Passive motion usually less painful than active motion.

▶ **Treatment options**
Conservative: Passive physical therapy • NSAIDs • Shoulder rest • Subacromial steroid injection.
Surgical: Expand subacromial space (acromioplasty).

▶ **Course and prognosis**
Without treatment, rotator cuff tear will usually develop.

▶ **What does the clinician want to know?**
Predisposing factors • Differential diagnoses.

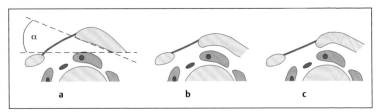

Fig. 8.8 a–c   Acromion shapes.
a Flat.
b Curved.
c Hooked.

Differential Diagnosis

(Sub-)luxation	– Contusions at typical sites
	– Hill–Sachs lesion
	– Labral lesions possible
Neoplasia	– Space-occupying mass
Cervical spine pathology	– Radiographs of cervical spine showing degenerative changes
Calcific tendonitis	– Calcium deposits

Tips and Pitfalls

Failure to clarify cervical spine changes.

Selected References

Fritz RC. Magnetic resonance imaging of sports-related injuries to the shoulder: impingement and rotator cuff. Radiol Clin North Am 2002; 40: 217–234

Koester MC, George MS, Kuhn JE. Shoulder impingement syndrome. Am J Med 2005; 118: 452–455

Neer CS. Impingement lesions. Clin Orthop 1983; 173: 70–77

Definition

▶ **Epidemiology**
10% of all fractures ● Age predilection: 50% in children under 10 years of age, and 70% in people up to age 40.

▶ **Etiology, pathophysiology, pathogenesis**
Indirect trauma, e.g., fall onto the shoulder or outstretched arm ● Rarely direct trauma (fall or blow to the shoulder) ● Perinatal.

Imaging Signs

▶ **Modality of choice**
Radiographs in two planes ● PA view and images with 30° cephalad angulation.

▶ **Radiographic/CT findings**
In fractures of the middle third of the clavicle, often bending wedge as well as posterocranial displacement of the medial fragment and mediocaudal displacement of the lateral fragment.
Allman classification of fracture location:
– Middle third of clavicle: shaft fractures ● 80%.
– Acromial third of clavicle: lateral fractures ● 15%.
– Sternal third of clavicle: medial fractures ● 5%.
Neer subclassification of acromial fractures:
– Type I: more common ● Lateral to coracoclavicular ligaments ● Stable.
– Type II: medial fragment no longer stabilized by coracoclavicular ligaments ● Displacement ● Risk of pseudarthrosis ● Unstable.
The Orthopedic Trauma Association (OTA) provides an alternative fracture classification.

Clinical Aspects

▶ **Typical presentation**
Pain ● Swelling ● Hematoma ● Malalignment ● Crepitation.

▶ **Treatment options**
Usually conservative with a sling ● Operative management with plate fixation and/or tension-band wiring ● Surgical indications: open fracture, significant displacement (greater than shaft width), interposed fragment, associated injuries, displaced lateral fracture.

▶ **Course and prognosis**
Usually good prognosis ● Average time to consolidation is 2–3 weeks in children and 4 weeks in adults.
Complications: pseudarthrosis ● Secondary displacement ● Related neurovascular injuries (brachial plexus, subclavian artery and vein).

▶ **What does the clinician want to know?**
Classification of fracture type ● Displacement ● Intermediate fragment.

Fig. 9.1 a, b
Clavicle fracture.
a PA radiograph of the left clavicle in a 50-year-old man who had fallen off a bicycle. Segmental fracture of the middle third of the clavicle with an intermediate fragment and elevation of the medial clavicle due to the pulling action of the sternocleidomastoid muscle.
b Follow-up radiograph after reduction and plate fixation.

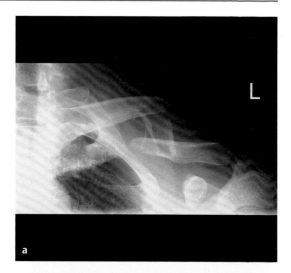

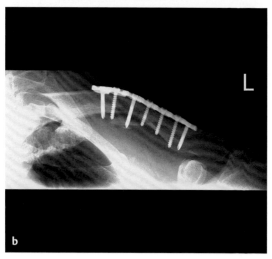

Differential Diagnosis

Acromioclavicular dislocation (Tossy) – No fracture
  – Widened acromioclavicular joint gap

Tips and Pitfalls

Missing a nondisplaced fracture of the middle third of the clavicle due to superimposed first rib • Missing a fracture of the sternal third when there is no or only minimal displacement (costoclavicular ligament) with superimposed vertebrae and ribs • Confusing clavicle fracture with sternoclavicular joint injury or nonossified epiphyseal growth plate (which is open medially up to age 22).

Selected References

Kumar R, Madewell JE, Swischuk LE, Lindell MM, David R. The clavicle: normal and abnormal. Radiographics 1989; 9(4): 677–706

Prescher A. Anatomical basics, variations, and degenerative changes of the shoulder joint and shoulder girdle [review]. Eur J Radiol 2000; 35(2): 88–102

Ridpath CA, Wilson AJ. Shoulder and humerus trauma [review]. Semin Musculoskelet Radiol 2000; 4(2): 151–170

Definition

Synonym: Tossy injury
▶ **Epidemiology**
12 % of all separations involving the shoulder girdle ● Men are affected 5–10 times as often as women ● Age predilection: 60 % of all patients are under age 40.
▶ **Etiology, pathophysiology, pathogenesis**
Direct trauma from blow to the acromion; less often indirect trauma (fall onto flexed elbow). Injury of the capsule and ACJ ligaments: acromioclavicular ligament and coracoclavicular ligament (consists of trapezoid and conoid ligaments).

Imaging Signs

▶ **Modality of choice**
Radiographs: AP views and views with 15° cephalad angulation ● After excluding lateral clavicle fracture, stress view with 5- to 10-kg weights on both sides.
▶ **Radiographic findings**
Size of joint space, comparing injured and uninjured sides ● Coracoclavicular distance (normal: 1–1.3 cm) and acromioclavicular distance (normal: 0.3–0.8 cm), comparing sides ● Step-off between acromion and clavicle.
Tossy classification:
– Tossy I: ACJ capsule distention with sprained acromioclavicular ligament ● No radiographic signs, but considerable pain or slightly widened joint space (compare with contralateral side).
– Tossy II: rupture of acromioclavicular ligament and partial tear or sprain of coracoclavicular ligament ● Radiographs show widening of ACJ space to 1–1.5 cm ● High clavicle, elevated as much as half the width of the shaft (25–50 % compared to uninjured side).
– Tossy III: rupture of both ligaments ● Acromioclavicular joint space on radiographs > 1.5 cm ● Clavicle elevated by over half the width of the shaft (> 50 % compared to uninjured side).
Rockwood classification:
– Rockwood I–III correspond to Tossy I–III.
– Rockwood IV: posterior displacement of clavicle with trapezius injury ● Variably large ACJ space.
– Rockwood V: extreme cephalad displacement of the clavicle (more than twice the width of the shaft) and soft-tissue injury.
– Rockwood VI: displacement of lateral portion of clavicle to below the acromion.

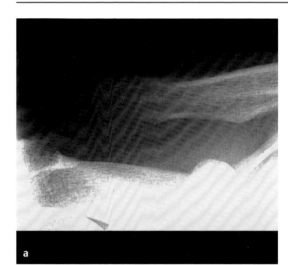

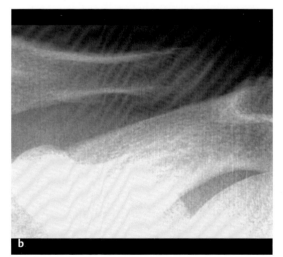

Fig. 9.2 a, b Separation of acromioclavicular joint (Tossy II). A 33-year-old man with ACJ pain after falling onto his elbow. PA radiograph of right ACJ (**a**) as well as contralateral side (**b**) for comparison. Separation of the right ACJ and elevation of the clavicle by nearly half the width of the shaft (Tossy II). The acromioclavicular joint space measures 1.2 cm (normal: maximum 0.8 cm).

Fractures and Dislocations

Fig. 9.3 Separation of acromioclavicular joint (Tossy III) in a 27-year-old man who had fallen off a bicycle. ACJ separation with clavicle elevated by twice the width of the shaft (Tossy III).

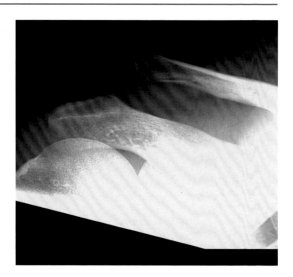

Clinical Aspects

▶ **Typical presentation**

Swelling ● Pain on pressure over the ACJ ● Step-off ("piano key") with clavicle elevation.

Complications: soft-tissue injuries ● Persistently elevated clavicle ● Pain ● Limited range of motion ● Instability after conservative management.

▶ **Treatment options**

– Tossy I–II: conservative with Desault or Gilchrist bandage.

– Tossy III: in athletic patients, ligament suture and reinforcement with resorbable polydioxanone S (PDS) cord ● Conservative treatment is a possible alternative.

– Rockwood IV–V: surgical management.

▶ **Course and prognosis**

Usually good functional result after conservative and surgical management.

▶ **What does the clinician want to know?**

Width of ACJ space compared to uninjured side ● Coracoclavicular distance compared to uninjured side ● Elevated clavicle.

Differential Diagnosis

Clavicle fracture	– Fracture line

Fractures and Dislocations

Tips and Pitfalls

Misdiagnosing lateral clavicle fracture (epiphysiolysis) in children as ACJ separation ● Misinterpretation due to individual variability of joint appearance and when stress radiographs are omitted ● Missing acromioclavicular separation on AP views in patients with posterior dislocation of the lateral end of the clavicle without cephalad displacement (Rockwood IV).

Selected References

Antonio GE, Cho JH, Chung CB, Trudell DJ, Resnick D. Pictorial essay. MR imaging appearance and classification of acromioclavicular joint injury. AJR Am J Roentgenol 2003; 180(4): 1103–1110

Keats TE, Pope TL Jr. The acromioclavicular joint: normal variation and the diagnosis of dislocation. Skeletal Radiol 1988; 17(3): 159–162

Vanarthos WJ, Ekman EF, Bohrer SP. Radiographic diagnosis of acromioclavicular joint separation without weight bearing: importance of internal rotation of the arm. AJR Am J Roentgenol 1994; 162(1): 120–122

Definition

▶ **Epidemiology**
4–5% of all fractures • Predominantly occur in older patients.

▶ **Etiology, pathophysiology, pathogenesis**
Trauma usually minimal • Fall onto an outstretched arm or direct blow to the lateral aspect of the humerus (often with osteoporosis) • In younger patients, more severe trauma is needed and displaced fractures or fracture-dislocations are more common.

Imaging Signs

▶ **Modality of choice**
Radiography • CT.

▶ **Radiographic/CT findings**
Radiograph of the shoulder joint in two planes (AP and transthoracic or Y-view) • Perhaps axial view to evaluate lesser tubercle • Modified Neer classification based on number of fragments and malalignment of four main segments (humeral head epiphysis, humerus metaphysis/diaphysis (surgical neck), and lesser and greater tubercles) • Displacement is diagnosed on the basis of 1 cm or more displacement or 45° angulation.
  – Neer 1: nondisplaced fracture of one or more fragments.
  Displaced fractures:
  – Neer 2: fracture of the anatomical neck, two-fragment fracture, one displaced fragment.
  – Neer 3: fracture of the surgical neck, two-fragment fracture, one displaced fragment.
  – Neer 4: fracture of the greater tubercle, without or with additional fracture of the surgical neck or lesser tubercle; two- to four-fragment fracture, up to three displaced fragments possible.
  – Neer 5: fracture of the lesser tubercle, two- to four-fragment fracture.
  – Neer 6: fracture-dislocations.
  AO classification scheme provides an alternative system.

▶ **CT findings**
Imaging of joint involvement, fragments, and displacement without superimpositions.

Clinical Aspects

▶ **Typical presentation**
Pain • Swelling • Limited range of motion after fall onto arm. • Humeral head necrosis, especially in fractures with three or four fragments and in fractures involving the anatomic neck (13–34%) • Post-traumatic shoulder stiffness • Omarthritis • Rotator cuff tear • Nerve damage (axillary nerve) • Vascular injuries (axillary artery, 5% in displaced fractures).

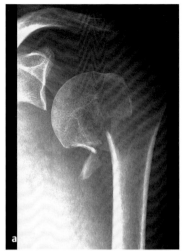

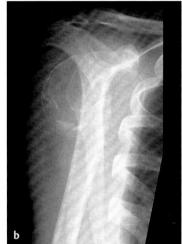

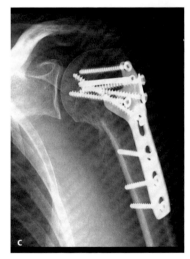

Fig. 9.4 a–c Subcapital fracture of the humerus in a 65-year-old woman after falling onto her outstretched hand.
a AP view and **b** Y-view of the shoulder. Subcapital fracture of the humerus with separation of a wedge-shaped fragment. Inferoposterior displacement of the humeral head (Neer III). The greater and lesser tubercles are intact.
c Follow-up radiograph after reduction and plate fixation.

▶ **Treatment options**

Goal: early mobilization given risk of capsule atrophy • Conservative treatment (Gilchrist bandage) for two-fragment fractures and nondisplaced or minimally displaced fractures • Surgery: plate fixation or fixed-angle proximal humerus nail, if needed with cerclage wiring of the tubercles (if displacement of greater tubercle exceeds 5 mm) • Endoprosthesis mainly in older patients with fractures involving four or more fragments and omarthritis.

Neer 1

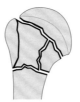

Nondisplaced or
minimally displaced

Neer 2
Anatomical
neck

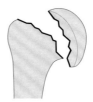

2-segment fracture

Neer 3
Surgical
neck

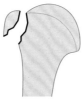 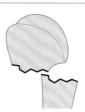 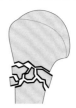

2-segment fracture
with axial displacement

2-segment fracture
with lateral displacement

Comminuted
fracture

Neer 4
Greater
tubercle

 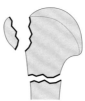 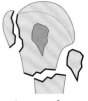

2-segment fracture

3-segment fracture
(combined with
surgical neck fracture)

4-segment fracture
(combined with
surgical neck and
lesser tubercle fractures)

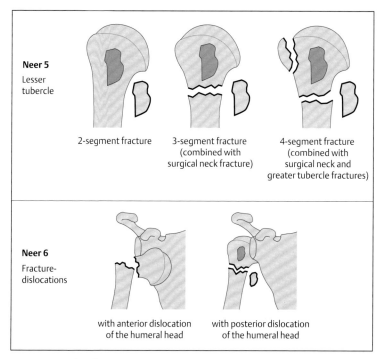

Neer 5
Lesser
tubercle

2-segment fracture

3-segment fracture
(combined with
surgical neck fracture)

4-segment fracture
(combined with
surgical neck and
greater tubercle fractures)

Neer 6
Fracture-
dislocations

with anterior dislocation
of the humeral head

with posterior dislocation
of the humeral head

Fig. 9.5 Neer classification.

▶ **Course and prognosis**
Good prognosis in impacted fractures with minimal displacement ● Prognosis worsens with the number of fragments (humeral head necrosis, arthritis).

▶ **What does the clinician want to know?**
Number of fragments ● Displacement involving joint ● Angulation of the humeral head ● Involvement of greater tubercle?

Tips and Pitfalls

Missing avulsion of greater or lesser tubercle.

Selected References

Helmy N, Hintermann B. New trends in the treatment of proximal humerus fractures [review]. Clin Orthop Relat Res 2006; 442: 100–108

Nho SJ, Brophy RH, Barker JU, Cornell CN, MacGillivray JD. Innovations in the management of displaced proximal humerus fractures [review]. J Am Acad Orthop Surg 2007; 15(1): 12–26

Sanchez-Sotelo J. Proximal humerus fractures [review]. Clin Anat 2006; 19(7): 588–598

Definition

▶ **Epidemiology**
Most common type of dislocation ● 50% of all dislocations involving the large joints ● Incidence is 15 in 100 000.

▶ **Etiology, pathophysiology, pathogenesis**
Predisposing factors include poorly centered humerus head in the bony socket ● Causes: usually traumatic, less often habitual with capsule laxity.
Types of dislocation:
– Anterior dislocation (97%): usually due to indirect application of force ● Combination of extension, external rotation, and abduction.
– Posterior dislocation (2–3%): usually due to indirect forces ● Flexion, internal rotation, and adduction, e.g., in electric shock injuries or epileptic seizure.
– Rare types: dislocation with separation of the roof of the shoulder joint ● Inferior dislocation (luxatio erecta).

Imaging Signs

▶ **Modality of choice**
Radiographs.

▶ **Radiographic findings**
Radiographs in two planes: AP tangential view of glenoid cavity, and trans-scapular view.
Anterior dislocation: Humeral head lies anteroinferiorly, usually below the coracoid process ● In rare situations, it may be caught on the inferior border of the glenoid cavity.
Posterior dislocation: Humeral head overlapping border of the glenoid cavity ● Joint space cannot be visualized.
Commonly associated injuries:
– Avulsion of the greater tubercle.
– Hill–Sachs lesion: anterior dislocation with an osseous defect on the posterolateral humeral head ● Corresponds to the site where the humeral head was caught on the inferior border of the glenoid cavity ● Possible AP view with internal rotation of the arm.
– Reverse Hill–Sachs defect: occurs in posterior shoulder joint dislocation ● Near the lesser tubercle.
– Bankart lesion: cartilaginous and/or osseous defect on the inferior border of the glenoid cavity/labrum.

▶ **CT findings**
CT especially if Bankart lesion is suspected ● Perhaps CT arthrography: intra-articular air insufflation under direct visualization, imaging of the labrum, joint capsule, and glenohumeral ligaments.

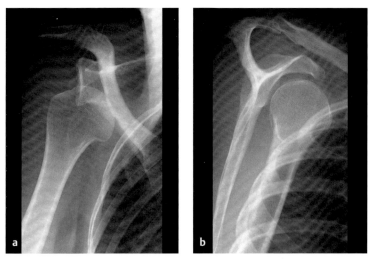

Fig. 9.6 a, b Anterior shoulder joint dislocation in a 46-year-old woman after falling onto her outstretched arm. **a** AP radiograph of right shoulder joint, with the contralateral side of the body rotated 40° anteriorly, and **b** Y-view. The articular fossa is empty. Anteroinferior dislocation of the humeral head to below the coracoid process.

▶ **MRI findings**
Method of choice for imaging suspected labral lesions, capsular ligament lesions, and rotator cuff lesions • MR arthrography: inject a mixture of gadolinium (Gd) and iodine-containing contrast agent • Dilution: NaCl–Gd mixture = 1 : 200, iodine-containing contrast agent 1 : 1.

Clinical Aspects
. . . .

▶ **Typical presentation**
Pain • Limited range of motion • Shoulder slightly abducted in anteroinferior dislocation.

▶ **Treatment options**
Closed reduction after administration of muscle relaxants and analgesics, or if necessary, under short-acting narcotic • Open reduction: if closed reduction under anesthesia fails, or with additional fracture • Capsule tightening if recurrent dislocations • Reattachment in Bankart lesions.

▶ **Course and prognosis**
Potential for recurrent dislocation with capsular damage arising from post-traumatic dislocation, especially in younger patients • Very rarely, axillary nerve or artery injury • Rotator cuff tear, mostly in patients over age 40.

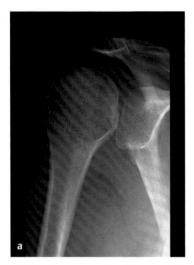 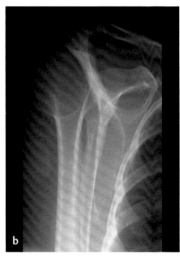

Fig. 9.7 a, b Posterior shoulder joint dislocation in a 45-year-old woman who fell off a bicycle.
a Radiograph of the right shoulder joint. The joint space cannot be visualized on the AP view; the arm is rotated medially.
b Y-view clearly demonstrates posterior dislocation.

▶ **What does the clinician want to know?**
Direction of dislocation • Associated fracture • Hill–Sachs lesion • Bankart lesion • Proper articulation after reduction.

Tips and Pitfalls
....

Missing a posterior shoulder dislocation, especially if no tangential view is taken to visualize the glenoid cavity • Missing associated bony or labral injury (CT!).

Selected References

Ly JQ, Beall DP, Sanders TG. MR imaging of glenohumeral instability. AJR Am J Roentgenol 2003; 181(1): 203–213
Stiles RG, Otte MT. Imaging of the shoulder [review]. Radiology. 1993; 188(3): 603–613
Woertler K, Waldt S. MR imaging in sports-related glenohumeral instability [review]. Eur Radiol 2006; 16(12): 2622–2636

Definition

▶ **Epidemiology**
Manifestation between ages 20–60 (85% of cases) ● Women affected twice as often as men ● Most common elbow fracture in adults ● Second most common elbow fracture (after supracondylar humerus fracture) in children.

▶ **Etiology, pathophysiology, pathogenesis**
Fall onto the outstretched hand, direct blow to the elbow. In 30% of cases associated bone and soft-tissue injuries (collateral ligament lesion, damage to the articular disk of distal radioulnar joint).

Imaging Signs

▶ **Modality of choice**
Radiography ● CT in uncertain fractures, e.g., in radiographically detectable joint effusion (positive fat pad sign).

▶ **Radiographic findings**
AP and true lateral views ● Radial head–capitellum view ● Radiolucent line on radial head ● Compression fracture ● Sagittal fracture through radial head and neck (chisel fracture) ● Extra-articular fracture involving only the neck ● Comminuted fracture ● Discreet fractures may be visible only as fine radiodense lines with associated effusion ● Displacement exceeding 1–2 mm or 20° angulation.
Mason classification system:
  – Type I: nondisplaced fracture of articular surface or neck.
  – Type II: displaced fracture (with impaction or angulation) involving more than 30% of the radial head.
  – Type III: comminuted fracture.
  – Type IV: radial head fracture with dislocation of the radial head.
Essex–Lopresti fracture: Comminuted fracture of the radial head ● Shortening of the radial shaft ● Instability, subluxation, or dislocation of distal radioulnar joint ● Interosseous membrane rupture.

▶ **CT findings**
CT indicated in comminuted fractures or indeterminate radiographic findings ● Evaluation of fragment position ● Determine degree of dislocation.

Fig. 9.8 a, b   Radial head fracture in a 32-year-old man who fell off a bicycle.

a Lateral radiograph showing a positive fat pad sign consistent with joint effusion. No visible fracture line.

b Sagittal reconstruction of axial thin-slice (1 mm) CT images of the elbow joint. Chisel fracture of the radial head and intra-articular step-off.

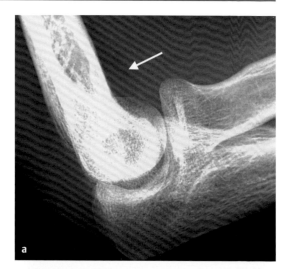

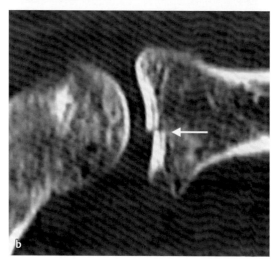

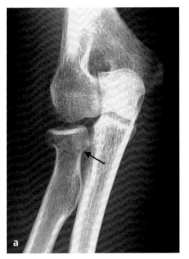
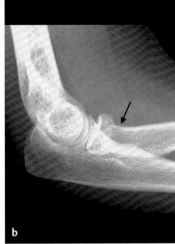

Fig. 9.9 a, b Radial head fracture in a 29-year-old woman who fell onto her outstretched hand while in-line skating.
a AP radiograph showing radiolucent line on the radial head.
b Lateral radiograph. No joint effusion in the extra-articular fracture.

Clinical Aspects

▶ **Typical presentation**
Pain over the radius on palpation ● Favoring ● Hematoma ● Pronation/supination impossible.

▶ **Treatment options**
Nondisplaced fractures are treated conservatively with a plaster splint/cast for 14 days, followed by early motion therapy ● Displaced (< 2 mm) fracture-dislocations are treated with open reduction of fragments ● If attempted reduction fails in comminuted fractures, management with resection or radial head prosthesis.

▶ **Course and prognosis**
Consolidation after 6–8 weeks.

▶ **What does the clinician want to know?**
Fracture classification ● Position/displacement ● Dislocation ● Size of intra-articular step-off ● Associated injuries (humeral head or coronoid process) ● Signs of capsular ligament injuries (cortical avulsion at epicondylar ligament attachment site).

Differential Diagnosis
....

Monteggia fracture   – Radial head dislocation with proximal ulnar fracture

Tips and Pitfalls
....

Missing a fracture on conventional radiographs in two planes (fat pad sign!) ● Radial head view is mandatory in suspected fractures—CT should be obtained if findings still negative but patient has suggestive pain on palpation.

Selected References

Cunningham PM. MR imaging of trauma: elbow and wrist [review]. Semin Musculoskelet Radiol 2006; 10(4): 284–292

Kaplan LJ, Potter HG. MR imaging of ligament injuries to the elbow. Radiol Clin North Am 2006; 44(4): 583–594, ix

O'Driscoll SW, Jupiter JB, Cohen MS, Ring D, McKee MD. Difficult elbow fractures: pearls and pitfalls. Instr Course Lect 2003; 52: 113–134

Roidis NT, Papadakis SA, Rigopoulos N, et al. Current concepts and controversies in the management of radial head fractures. Orthopedics 2006; 29(10): 904–916

Sonin A. Fractures of the elbow and forearm. Semin Musculoskelet Radiol 2000; 4(2): 171–191

Definition

▶ **Epidemiology**
In children the supracondylar humerus fracture is the most common (60%) fracture involving the elbow • Lateral condyle fractures (15%) are the second most common, followed by medial epicondylar fractures (10%) • Usually in children age 3–10 • Peak incidence: age 5–8.

▶ **Etiology, pathophysiology, pathogenesis**
In contrast to supracondylar and epicondylar humerus fractures, condylar fractures are intra-articular fractures • Most condylar fractures cross the epiphyseal plate • Involvement of ossific nucleus of humeral head is rare • Greatest fracture tendency is between ages 7 and 10 due to inadequate stability of immature bone, whereas at older ages dislocation is more common • Divided into fractures of the radial and ulnar condyles and transcondylar fractures (very rare).

Imaging Signs

▶ **Modality of choice**
Radiography.

▶ **Radiographic findings**
Views of the elbow in two planes • Radiographs of contralateral side generally not part of routine work-up • On lateral views, the fracture line runs from posteroproximal to anterodistal and terminates at or crosses the epiphyseal plate • On AP views, the fracture line runs from the proximal periphery to the distal, central portion of the bone • Impossible to distinguish between a fracture that is incomplete and stable versus one that is complete and unstable, dividing the epiphysis • Distinction is usually made after a few days once displacement occurs (unstable) or does not occur (stable) in the cast • Displacement: fragment gap exceeding 2 mm • Indirect fracture signs: effusion and positive fat pad sign.

Clinical Aspects

▶ **Typical presentation**
Severe swelling • Deformity • Severe pain • Limited range of motion.

▶ **Treatment options**
Reduction under general anesthesia • In nondisplaced fractures, conservative treatment: long arm cast for 4 weeks • In displaced fractures, operative treatment: metaphyseal compression screw fixation.

▶ **Course and prognosis**
Good prognosis in nondisplaced fractures • Delayed healing or pseudarthrosis possible in unstable or displaced fractures.

▶ **What does the clinician want to know?**
Path of fracture line • Fragment displacement.

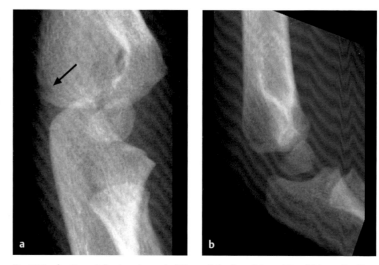

Fig. 9.10 a, b Recent fracture (arrow) of the radial epicondyle. **a** AP and **b** lateral radiographs of the elbow joint.

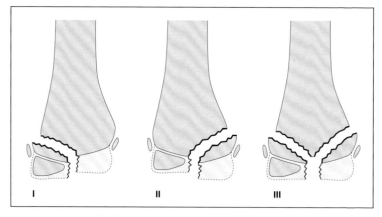

Fig. 9.11 Intra-articular fractures of the distal humerus. Radial condyle (I), ulnar condyle (II), and transcondylar fractures (III).

Differential Diagnosis

Supracondylar fracture   – On lateral views fracture is proximal to the epiphyseal plate

Tips and Pitfalls

Missing a nondisplaced fracture.

Selected References

Hammond WA, Kay RM, Skaggs DL. Supracondylar humerus fractures in children. AORN J 1998; 68(2): 186–199

Kocher MS, Waters PM, Micheli LJ. Upper extremity injuries in the paediatric athlete. Sports Med 2000; 30(2): 117–135

Lins RE, Simovitch RW, Waters PM. Pediatric elbow trauma. Orthop Clin North Am 1999; 30(1): 119–132

Definition

▶ **Epidemiology**
Most common fracture occurring in humans ● 25% of all fractures ● Incidence is 200–300 in 100 000 ● Peak incidence: age 6–10 and 60–70 (osteoporosis).

▶ **Etiology, pathophysiology, pathogenesis**
 – Extension fracture (Colles fracture): most common type ● Fall onto dorsiflexed hand ● Dorsal displacement of the distal fragment.
 – Flexion fracture (Smith fracture): less common ● Fall onto palmar-flexed hand ● Palmar displacement of the distal fragment.
 – Fracture-dislocation (Galeazzi): fracture of distal radius shaft ● Dislocation of distal ulnar head ● Distal forearm completely unstable.

Imaging Signs

▶ **Modality of choice**
Radiography ● In fractures with displacement, possibly preoperative CT for precise depiction of fracture line ● MRI when radiographically occult fracture is suspected.

▶ **Radiographic findings**
Wrist radiographs in two planes (DP and lateral).
Frykman classification (of Colles fractures):
 – Grade I: extra-articular distal radius fracture.
 – Grade II: grade I plus ulnar styloid process fracture.
 – Grade III: involvement of radiocarpal joint.
 – Grade IV: grade III plus ulnar styloid process fracture.
 – Grade V: involvement of radioulnar joint.
 – Grade VI: grade V plus ulnar styloid process fracture.
 – Grade VII: involvement of both joints.
 – Grade VIII: grade VII plus ulnar styloid process fracture.
AO classification provides an alternative system.
Special types of distal radius fracture:
 – Chauffeur fracture (Hutchinson fracture): avulsion of the ulnar styloid process ● Sagittal fracture line.
 – Reverse Hutchinson fracture: avulsion of the ulnar margin of the radial articular surface.
 – Barton fracture: avulsion of the posterior margin of the radius ● Coronal fracture line.
 – Reverse Barton fracture: avulsion of the anterior margin of the radius.
 – Die-punch fracture: circumscribed depression of the lunate facet of the radial articular surface.
 – Galeazzi fracture-dislocation: fracture of the distal radius shaft and dislocation of the distal ulnar head.

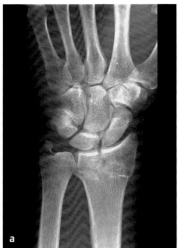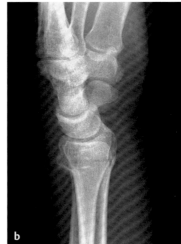

Fig. 9.12 a, b AP (**a**) and lateral (**b**) views of the wrist joint in a 55-year-old man after falling onto his outstretched hand. Distal radius fracture at a typical site (Colles fracture), involving the radiocarpal and radioulnar joints and avulsion of the ulnar styloid process. The radial articular surface is tilted about 12° posteriorly. Frykman type VIII fracture.

Clinical Aspects

▶ **Typical presentation**
Tenderness ● Soft-tissue swelling ● Limited wrist motion ● Malalignment.

▶ **Treatment options**
Conservative treatment: Possible in 90% of distal radius fractures ● Important: regular follow-up radiographs to detect for recurrent displacement.
Surgical treatment: Open fractures ● Irreducible displacement ● Unstable fractures: avulsion of the ulnar styloid process, Smith fracture, dorsal intra-articular fractures, comminuted fractures ● Procedures: Kirschner wiring, plate fixation, external fixation.

▶ **Course and prognosis**
Complications: despite casting, secondary displacement may occur up to 2 weeks after reduction ● Sudeck atrophy ● Post-traumatic carpal tunnel syndrome ● Post-traumatic arthritis ● Scapholunate ligament lesion with carpal instability.

▶ **What does the clinician want to know?**
Path of fracture line ● Involvement of articular surfaces ● Avulsion of ulnar styloid process (hence unstable fracture requiring operative treatment) ● Displacement ● Impaction ● Dislocated radius or ulna ● Ulna-plus condition ● Any additional injuries (scaphoid fracture, dislocations of carpal bones, scapholunate lig-

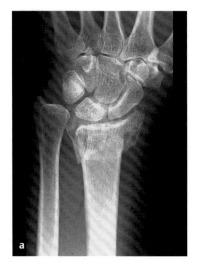 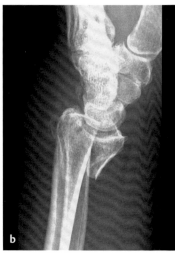

Fig. 9.13 a, b AP (**a**) and lateral (**b**) views of the wrist joint in a 54-year-old woman who fell onto her hand in palmar flexion. Smith fracture with comminution of the radial articular surface. Palmar displacement of impacted fracture fragments and ulna-plus condition. Additional triquetral fracture (**b**).

ament lesion) • Inclination of the radial articular surface (normal palmar tilt is 10–12° on lateral views and normal ulnar angulation of radial articular surface is 15–25° on AP views).

Tips and Pitfalls

Missing occult fractures on radiographs (cross-sectional imaging!) • Missing associated injuries (e.g., scapholunate ligament lesions or triquetral fracture).

Selected References

Cunningham PM. MR imaging of trauma: elbow and wrist. Semin Musculoskelet Radiol 2006; 10(4): 284–292

Handoll HH, Madhok R, Howe TE. Rehabilitation for distal radial fractures in adults. Cochrane Database Syst Rev 2006 Jul 19; 3: CD003324

Lichtman DM, Joshi A. Acute injuries of the distal radioulnar joint and triangular fibrocartilage complex. Instr Course Lect 2003; 52: 175–183

Ruch DS, Weiland AJ, Wolfe SW, et al. Current concepts in the treatment of distal radial fractures. Instr Course Lect 2004; 53: 389–401

Steinbach LS, Smith DK. MRI of the wrist. Clin Imaging 2000; 24: 298–322

Definition

Synonym: Navicular fracture

▶ **Epidemiology**

Most common fracture involving the carpal bones (50–80%) ● Peak incidence: age 10–40.

▶ **Etiology, pathophysiology, pathogenesis**

Usually due to indirect trauma ● Fall onto extended (dorsiflexed) hand in ulnar or radial abduction ● Additional load transference from the thumb or ball of the thumb ● Indirect trauma less common.

Classified by fracture plane or site:

- Boehler classification: transverse fracture (60%), horizontal oblique fracture (35%), vertical oblique fracture (3%).
- Proximal third (20–30%), middle third (60–80%), distal third (rare, but with better tendency to heal since blood supply is from distal).

Imaging Signs

▶ **Modality of choice**

Radiographs ● If there is clinical suspicion, but radiographic findings are unremarkable, perhaps CT or MRI.

▶ **Radiographic findings**

Radiographs of the wrist in two planes ● "Scaphoid quartet" (four planes) ● Stress views with hand in ulnar abduction and positioning the scaphoid parallel to the film (lifting the radial side of the hand about 40°) ● Often difficult to detect, especially nondisplaced fractures, incomplete fractures near the tubercle, and small avulsion fractures ● Radiolucent line with cortical interruption.

Signs of instability:

- Fragment displacement exceeding 1 mm.
- Signs of ligamentous lesion, e.g., scapholunate dissociation (scapholunate gap > 2 mm) and dorsal intercalated segment instability (DISI) (scapholunate angle > 60°).
- Humpback deformity: angulation of the scaphoid toward the fracture line; associated with significantly worsened chances of consolidation.
- Pseudarthrosis/nonunion.

Radiographic signs of pseudarthrosis: resorption zones and cysts along the band-like and indistinctly-bordered fracture gap ● Followed by sclerosis and filling in of the fracture surfaces with fibrous tissue.

▶ **CT findings**

More sensitive than radiography ● Fragment position ● Fracture lines ● Displacement ● Follow-up of healing process with depiction of callus formation or resorption zones and marginal sclerosis.

▶ **MRI findings**

MRI if there is clinical suspicion despite negative radiographic findings ● Evaluation of associated capsular ligament injuries ● Useful for diagnosis of bone vitality ● Fracture line on T1-weighted images presents as a band of decreased sig-

Fig. 9.14 a, b
Scaphoid fracture (middle third).
a Capitate superimposed. **b** The fracture line is better visualized with ulnar abduction and ulnar tilting of the surface of the wrist.

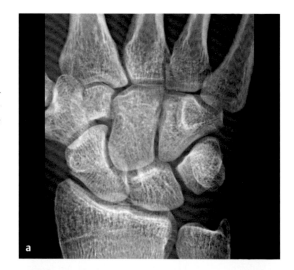

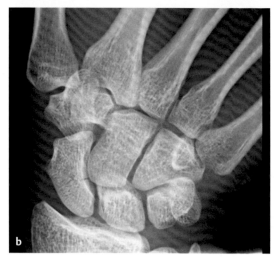

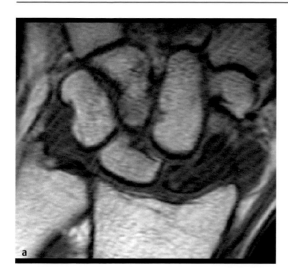

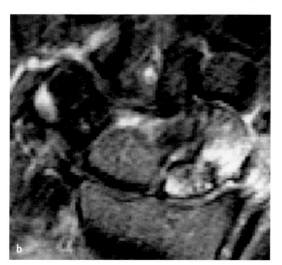

Fig. 9.15 a–d Scaphoid fracture. MRI.
a Noncontrast T1-weighted image showing extensive areas of decreased signal intensity.
b STIR image showing hyperintense signal with a hypointense fracture line.

c T1-weighted image after administration of contrast material. The proximal aspect of the scaphoid is nonenhancing, indicating disrupted blood supply and devitalization.

d Long-standing scaphoid necrosis with resorption of the proximal fragment as well as degenerative changes affecting the radiocarpal joint consistent with carpal instability and loss of carpal height.

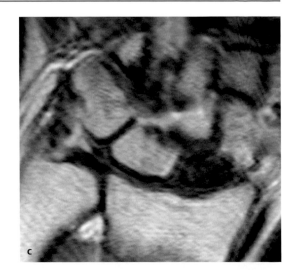

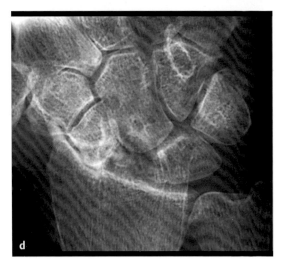

nal intensity • Band of increased signal intensity on T2-weighted images • In recent lesions, STIR and fat-saturated T2-weighted sequences provide sensitive depiction of marrow edema • False-positive results possible if there is diffusely decreased signal intensity on T1-weighted images without definitive detection of a fracture line.

Clinical Aspects

▶ **Typical presentation**
Tenderness over the anatomic snuffbox (radial fossa) • Loss of radial fossa contour • Pain with wrist motion.

▶ **Treatment options**
Conservative treatment: Stable fractures • Boehler cast (long arm cast including the metacarpophalangeal joints of the thumb and index finger for 4–6 weeks, followed by short arm cast for 4–6 weeks).
Surgical treatment: Unstable fractures • Reduction and screw fixation (Herbert screw) • Possible spongiosaplasty in delayed healing or pseudarthrosis • In pseudarthrosis, treatment with Matti-Russe I technique or, with nonunion defect, grafting after Russe II or Fisk–Hernandez • Postoperative long arm/short arm cast for 4–8 weeks.

▶ **Course and prognosis**
Heals only slowly • Tendency for nonunion • Necrosis of the scaphoid or part of it (usually proximal fragment) • Carpal instability.

▶ **What does the clinician want to know?**
Path of fracture line • Displacement • Evaluation of vitality/viability • Pseudarthrosis/nonunion.

Differential Diagnosis

| Bipartite scaphoid | – Rare |
| | – Already primarily rounded, sclerotic borders of bony elements |

Tips and Pitfalls

Missing the fracture.

Selected References

Dorsay TA, Major NM, Helms CA. Cost-effectiveness of immediate MR imaging versus traditional follow-up for revealing radiographically occult scaphoid fractures. AJR Am J Roentgenol 2001; 177(6): 1257–1263

Hunter D. Diagnosis and management of scaphoid fractures: a literature review. Emerg Nurse 2005; 13(7): 22–26

Definition

▶ **Epidemiology**
After scaphoid fracture, second most common fracture of the carpal bones (13%) ● Age predilection: young adults.

▶ **Etiology, pathophysiology, pathogenesis**
Axial compression trauma caused by a fall onto the hand ● Direct trauma ● In hyperextension trauma of the wrist, the triquetrum is compressed between the ulnar styloid process and the pisiform.

Imaging Signs

▶ **Modality of choice**
Radiographs of the wrist in two planes ● CT if radiographic findings equivocal.
Radiographic/CT findings
Dorsal avulsion fracture: In hyperextension of the wrist, bony avulsion of the radiotriquetral ligament or dorsal intercarpal ligament ● On lateral views, a small detached, dorsal fragment at the level of the triquetrum (usually not visible on AP views due to overlapping pisiform).
Fracture of triquetral body: Rare (3%) ● Radiolucent line in the triquetrum seen on AP views (usually not visible on lateral views since the lunate, capitate, and scaphoid overlap the triquetral body).

Clinical Aspects

▶ **Typical presentation**
Pain, especially with wrist flexion ● Pain and swelling over the ulnar dorsum of the hand distal to the ulnar styloid process ● Compression pain in the fourth and fifth digital rays ● Instability if accompanied by ligamentous rupture (on clinical examination) ● Complications: associated ligamentous injury may cause instability of the wrist joint ● Delayed sequela: carpal collapse.

▶ **Treatment options**
Usually plaster cast or splint immobilization for 2–4 weeks ● Operative treatment of displaced fractures.

▶ **Course and prognosis**
Triquetral fractures usually heal without sequelae.

▶ **What does the clinician want to know?**
Path of fracture line ● Displacement.

Tips and Pitfalls

Missing the fracture on radiography: it is often only detectable in one plane, and radiographic findings are often subtle ● Clinical examination of the patient is essential (palpation!).

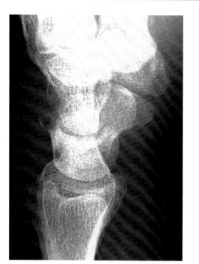

Fig. 9.16 Triquetral fracture in a 37-year-old man who fell onto his outstretched hand while in-line skating without a wrist guard. Lateral radiograph of the left wrist showing a dorsal avulsion fracture of the triquetrum.

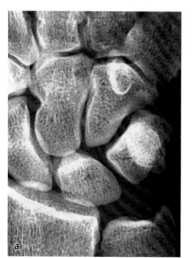

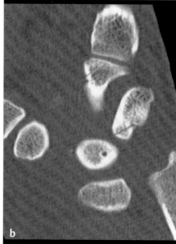

Fig. 9.17 a, b Triquetral fracture in a 31-year-old woman who fell onto her right hand while in-line skating without a wrist guard.

a AP view of the wrist showing a radiolucent line (fracture line) along the base of the triquetral body.

b CT, coronal reconstruction using 0.75-mm axial slices confirms the presence of a fracture.

Selected References

Geissler WB. Carpal fractures in athletes. Clin Sports Med 2001; 20(1): 167–188

Goldfarb CA, Yin Y, Gilula LA, Fisher AJ, Boyer MI. Wrist fractures: what the clinician wants to know. Radiology 2001; 219(1): 11–28

Miller RJ. Wrist MRI and carpal instability: what the surgeon needs to know, and the case for dynamic imaging. Semin Musculoskelet Radiol 2001; 5(3): 235–240

Schubert H. Triquetrum fracture. Can Fam Physician 2000; 46: 70–71

Definition

▶ **Epidemiology**
10% of all Alpine skiing injuries ● Also occurs in ice hockey and handball.

▶ **Etiology, pathophysiology, pathogenesis**
Thumb is caught on the grip or under the strap of the ski pole and forced dorsally and radially ● Ulnar collateral ligament rupture at the metacarpophalangeal joint of the thumb ● Interligamentous rupture or bony avulsion (more often distal than proximal) ● Complication possible when loose proximal end of the ligament is driven below the tendon aponeurosis of the adductor pollicis (Stener lesion), preventing healing and leading to development of chronic instability.

Imaging Signs

▶ **Modality of choice**
Radiography.

▶ **Radiographic findings**
Radiographs in two planes ● After fracture is ruled out, stress radiographs ● Then examination of both hands, comparing injured and uninjured sides ● Detached bony fragment ● Degree of joint opening (laxity) exceeding 28° or difference of at least 20° between injured and uninjured sides.

▶ **MRI findings**
MRI only when diagnosis is uncertain or if rupture is older ● Coronal and axial images using T1-weighted and fat-saturated T2-weighted sequences ● Disrupted ulnar collateral ligament ● Bony avulsion is possible ● Proximal end of ligament may be displaced (Stener lesion).

Clinical Aspects

▶ **Typical presentation**
Tenderness ● Soft-tissue swelling ● Hematoma ● There may be a limited range of motion.

▶ **Treatment options**
Incomplete ruptures of the ulnar collateral ligament are treated with immobilization of the MCP joint in a thumb splint for 4 weeks ● If rupture is complete or there is bony avulsion or a high level of suspicion of a Stener lesion, treatment is within the first 10 days with direct suture repair of the ligament ● In avulsion fractures, transosseous cerclage and pull-out suture or fixation (wires, screws, anchors).

▶ **Course and prognosis**
Untreated or inadequately managed injuries result in limited function (e.g., grasping a bottle is impossible) with chronic MCP instability ("floppy joint") and impaired function that may affect the entire hand.

▶ **What does the clinician want to know?**
Bone involvement ● Degree of joint opening (laxity).

Fig. 9.18 Pain involving the MCP joint of the thumb after forced abduction during a fall while skiing. DP radiograph shows avulsion of an elongated bony fragment from the ulnar side of the base of the proximal phalanx of the thumb.

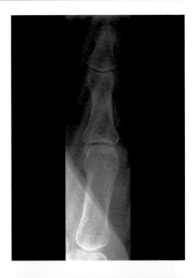

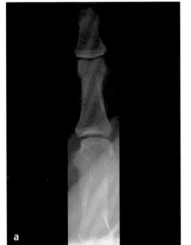

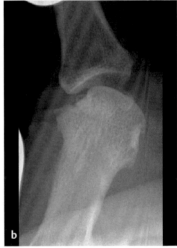

Fig. 9.19 a, b Fall while skiing with a ski pole in the hand.
a DP radiograph shows ossification on the radial aspect of the distal portion of the first metacarpal bone after earlier trauma. No recent fracture is detectable.
b View with radial abduction: 37° angulation in the MCP joint.

Differential Diagnosis

Fractures and/or dislocations of the phalanges and metacarpal bones are readily visualized on radiographs.

Tips and Pitfalls

On stress views, careful DP projection of the thumb MCP joint and correct positioning of the metacarpal bone against the proximal phalanx of the thumb are needed to produce sufficient stress to be evident radiographically.

Selected References

Newland CC. Gamekeeper's thumb. Orthop Clin North Am 1992; 23(1): 41–48

Spaeth HJ, Abrams RA, Bock GW, et al. Gamekeeper thumb: differentiation of nondisplaced and displaced tears of the ulnar collateral ligament with MR imaging. Work in progress. Radiology 1993; 188 (2): 553–556

Definition

▶ **Epidemiology**
11–13% of all fractures of the cervical spine • 1–2% of all vertebral fractures • Most common cervical spine injury in the elderly • Trauma-related injury that affects all age groups.

▶ **Etiology, pathophysiology, pathogenesis**
Usually hyperextension trauma.

Imaging Signs

▶ **Modality of choice**
Radiography is generally primary study • Radiographs of the cervical spine in two planes and odontoid view (horizontal beam with open mouth) • CT for visualization of C2 without superimposing structures.

▶ **Radiographic/CT findings**
Classification based on Anderson and D'Alonzo:
  – Type I: oblique fracture through the apex of the dens • Avulsion fracture of the alar ligaments • Stable • Very rare type of fracture.
  – Type II: transverse fracture through the base of the dens • Unstable • Most common type of fracture • With displacement, pseudarthrosis develops in 70%.
  – Type III: fracture through the body of the axis • Often anteroinferior displacement • Unstable • Tends not to develop pseudarthrosis.
Alternative classification of dens fractures based on AO system • Special variant: Hangman's fracture (bilateral fracture of C2 vertebral arch).

▶ **MRI findings**
MRI when neurologic deficit, spinal cord damage, or intraspinal hemorrhage is present.

Clinical Aspects

▶ **Typical presentation**
Neck pain • Painful restricted range of motion • Complications: paraplegia, pseudarthrosis, chronic pain syndrome, limited range of motion.

▶ **Treatment options**
Angulation of the dens or translation instability exceeding 2 mm requires urgent surgical management—risk of spinal cord compression!
  – Type I: without atlantoaxial instability, conservative treatment with rigid cervical collar for 4–6 weeks.
  – Type II: surgery if possible (e.g., closed reduction and anterior lag screw fixation) • If surgery is contraindicated and fracture is nondisplaced, halo traction for 12 weeks is possible • Conservative management often leads to pseudarthrosis.
  – Type III: halo fixation for 12 weeks • Usually heals completely.

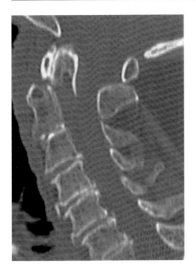

Fig. 9.20 A 91-year-old woman after a fall at home (forehead struck the wall). Sagittally reconstructed CT images reveal an unstable type II fracture of the dens with anterior displacement of the axis as well as the rest of the cervical spine.

▶ **Course and prognosis**
Prognosis usually good with surgical management and no primary neurologic dysfunction.

▶ **What does the clinician want to know?**
Fracture type according to Anderson and D'Alonzo classification • Stability • Displacement.

Differential Diagnosis

Os odontoideum	– Normal anatomic variant – Dens apophysis not fused with body of axis – Rounded with smooth contours
Persistent nonfusion	– In children – Fusion of os terminale with the body of axis occurs at age 11–12. Subdental synchondrosis may persist into adolescence (distinguish from type II fracture) – Fusion of posterior two anlagen of the arch of the atlas at age 2–3 – Fusion of posterior arch of atlas with axis in 7th year of life

Selected References

Bono CM, Vaccaro AR, Fehlings M, et al; Spine Trauma Study Group. Measurement techniques for upper cervical spine injuries: consensus statement of the Spine Trauma Study Group. Spine 2007; 32(5): 593–600

Deliganis AV, Baxter AB, Hanson JA, et al. Radiologic spectrum of craniocervical distraction injuries. Radiographics 2000; 20 (Spec No): S237–250. Erratum in: Radiographics 2001; 21(2): 520

Ellis GL. Imaging of the atlas (C1) and axis (C2). Emerg Med Clin North Am 1991; 9(4):719–732

Mirvis SE, Shanmuganathan K. Trauma radiology: Part V. Imaging of acute cervical spine trauma. J Intensive Care Med 1995; 10(1): 15–33

Definition

▶ **Epidemiology**
In the EU 414 000 cases per year, in Germany 100 000 ● Average age is 72 in men and 77 in women ● Affects women 2–3 times as often as men.

▶ **Etiology, pathophysiology, pathogenesis**
Usually medial fracture of the femoral neck (in 95 % fracture is intracapsular) ● Less often lateral fracture of the femoral neck (5 %) ● Typically caused by fall onto the hip with fracture of bones weakened by osteoporosis.

Imaging Signs

▶ **Modality of choice**
Radiography ● CT or MRI if radiographs equivocal.

▶ **Radiographic findings**
Hip radiographs in two planes (AP and axial views) ● Lauenstein view usually not possible due to pain ● Preoperative radiographs of whole pelvis to assess uninjured side (coxa vara/valga, length of femoral neck relative to ischial tuberosities) ● Radiolucent line through the femoral neck with or without fragment angulation.

Pauwels' classification is the most widely-used system, based on the angle of the fracture line to the horizontal plane:
– Type I: 30° angle to horizontal plane.
– Type II: 30–50° angle to horizontal plane.
– Type III: > 50° angle to horizontal plane.
Alternatively, AO or Garden's classification schemes may be used.

Clinical Aspects

▶ **Typical presentation**
Pain ● Externally rotated, shortened, and high-riding leg ● Hematoma ● Swelling.
Complications: Femoral head necrosis (10–20 %), especially in Pauwels type II and III fractures ● Delayed fracture healing or pseudarthrosis (5–25 %) ● Secondary coxarthrosis ● Risk of slippage, femoral head necrosis, and pseudarthrosis rises with increasing steepness of the fracture line.

▶ **Treatment options**
Conservative therapy is attempted in impacted type I Pauwels fractures and in valgus-producing abduction fractures ● Regular radiographic follow-up to monitor progression in order to detect displacement due to weight-bearing ● In Pauwels type II and III fractures in younger patients (< 65 years), cannulated screw fixation ● In older patients (especially with arthritis), endoprosthesis.

▶ **Course and prognosis**
Functional result primarily depends on overall health (comorbidities) of the patient ● Need for care often increases.

Fig. 9.21 A 70-year-old woman after a fall onto her left hip. AP radiograph of the left hip joint showing an impacted (abducted) medial femoral neck fracture (Pauwels type I–II) (34°, Garden type I). The fracture was stable and was therefore treated conservatively.

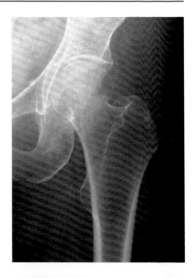

Fig. 9.22 A 62-year-old man who had fallen on his right hip. AP radiograph of the right hip joint showing a Pauwels type II displaced medial femoral neck fracture (61°). The fracture was unstable and was therefore managed surgically with cannulated screw fixation.

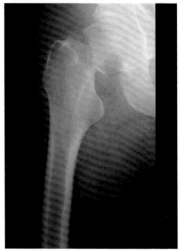

▶ **What does the clinician want to know?**

Degree of displacement (posterior angulation or vertical displacement of femoral head) ● Path of fracture line (grade) ● Impaction ● Coxarthrosis.

Differential Diagnosis

Peritrochanteric fracture	– Fracture line through the intertrochanteric region
Stress fracture	– Fatigue fracture due to overuse or insufficiency fracture in osteoporosis
	– Fracture line usually only faint, located medially in the cortex of the femoral neck with surrounding reactive sclerosis
	– Usually no recollection of significant trauma
Pathologic fracture	– Fracture arising from osteolysis

Tips and Pitfalls

The leg is held often in external rotation due to pain. On AP views in this position, the greater trochanter overlaps the femoral neck, making it possible to miss the fracture. If internal rotation of 15° cannot be achieved, the pelvis of the affected side should be supported by a cushion.

Selected References

Bartonicek J. Pauwels' classification of femoral neck fractures: correct interpretation of the original [review]. J Orthop Trauma 2001; 15(5): 358–360

Caviglia HA, Osorio PQ, Comando D. Classification and diagnosis of intracapsular fractures of the proximal femur [review]. Clin Orthop Relat Res 2002; (399): 17–27

Ohashi K, Brandser EA, el-Khoury GY. Role of MR imaging in acute injuries to the appendicular skeleton [review]. Radiol Clin North Am 1997; 35(3): 591–613

Schmidt AH, Swiontkowski MF. Femoral neck fractures. Orthop Clin North Am 2002; 33(1):97–111

Definition

▶ **Epidemiology**
40–45% of proximal femoral fractures ● As common as femoral neck fracture ● Average patient age is 70–80 years, somewhat older than in femoral neck fractures ● Women are affected 2–8 times as often as men.

▶ **Etiology, pathophysiology, pathogenesis**
Usually caused by a fall onto the hip ● Predilection for older patients whose bones are weakened by osteoporosis ● In younger patients, occurs only after severe trauma, e.g., snowboarding, in-line skating, or motorcycle accidents ● Fracture line usually runs diagonally from greater to lesser trochanter ● Rarely (10–15%) runs from lesser trochanter caudally and laterally (reverse pertrochanteric fracture).

Imaging Signs

▶ **Modality of choice**
Radiography: view of whole pelvis ● AP view of hip joint (depiction of proximal femoral shaft for implant placement) ● Axial view of hip joint with horizontal beam.

▶ **Radiographic findings**
Radiolucent line through intertrochanteric region ● There may be displacement and/or avulsion of the trochanters.
Evans classification scheme:
– Type I: nondisplaced ● Mostly stable ● Two fragments.
– Type II: displaced ● Small lesser trochanter fragment ● Intact medial cortex ● Reduction is possible given stable medial support.
– Type III: displaced ● Posteromedial comminuted area ● Irreducible ● Unstable.
– Type IV: comminuted fracture with additional greater trochanter fragment ● Lacking medial support after reduction ● Unstable.
– Type V: fracture line runs from proximal medial to distal lateral ("reverse oblique fracture").
There is an alternative AO classification system.

Clinical Aspects

▶ **Typical presentation**
Pain ● Externally rotated femur ● Shortened, high-riding leg ● Hematoma ● Swelling.

▶ **Treatment options**
Usually surgical treatment with Gamma nail, proximal femoral nail (permitting early weight bearing), or dynamic hip screw ● Endoprosthesis if coxarthrosis present.

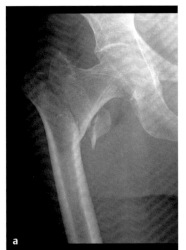 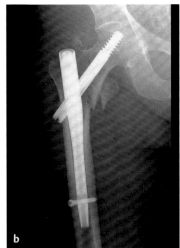

Fig. 9.23 a, b A 87-year-old woman who had fallen on her right side.
a AP radiograph of the right hip joint showing a pertrochanteric femoral fracture
with avulsion of the lesser trochanter and displacement (Evans type III).
b Postoperative follow-up radiograph after repair with a Gamma nail.

▶ **Course and prognosis**
Usually limited range of motion after surgery given patient age • Complications:
shaft fissure upon nail insertion • Migration of the femoral neck screw into the
joint • Delayed fracture healing or pseudarthrosis with subsequent material
breakage.

▶ **What does the clinician want to know?**
Path of fracture line • Involvement of lesser trochanter (lacking medial support) • Extent of concomitant coxarthrosis • Degree of displacement • Presence
of reverse pertrochanteric fracture (management of which is technically very
challenging).

Differential Diagnosis

Femoral neck fracture   – Fracture line in femoral neck (medial/lateral fracture)

Selected References

Shearman CM, el-Khoury GY. Pitfalls in the radiologic evaluation of extremity trauma:
part II. The lower extremity [review]. Am Fam Physician 1998; 57(6): 1314–1322

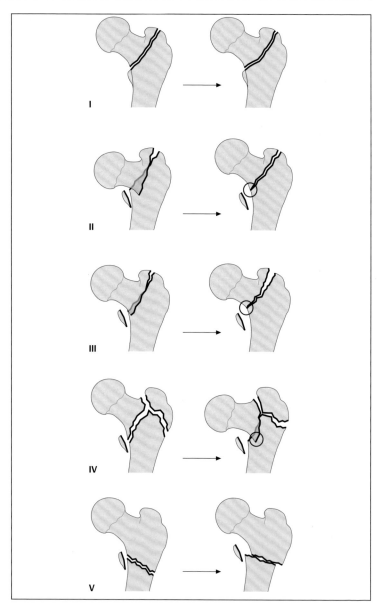

Fig. 9.24 Evans classification of fractures.

Definition

▶ **Epidemiology**
1% of all fractures.

▶ **Etiology, pathogenesis, pathophysiology**
Direct trauma: collision ("dashboard injury") or fall onto flexed knee • Indirect trauma (rare): sudden flexion with fully contracted quadriceps • Fracture in patellar resurfacing • Divided into transverse and oblique (60%; usually due to direct trauma), longitudinal (15%), multifragmentary (stellate or comminuted, 25%), and avulsion fractures of the superior or inferior patellar pole (due to direct or indirect trauma, often in children).

Imaging Signs

▶ **Modality of choice**
Radiography.

▶ **Radiographic findings**
AP and lateral views of the knee joint, tangential view of patella • Fracture line • Intra-articular loose bodies may be present • Patella baja if the quadriceps tendon is ruptured • Patella alta if the patellar tendon is ruptured.

▶ **CT findings**
CT only if there is discrepancy between radiographic findings and clinical presentation or if joint bodies are suspected.

▶ **MRI findings**
MRI if patellar dislocation (retinaculum) or patellar tendon/quadriceps tendon lesions are suspected • In patellar dislocation, contusions along inferomedial patella and inferolateral anterior border of the femoral condyle • Assessment of medial patellofemoral ligament (avulsion of patellar or femoral attachment) • Osteochondral fragments • Thickening • Disruption • Wavy appearance of fibers in quadriceps or patellar tendon rupture.

Clinical Aspects

History of trauma • Soft-tissue swelling • Palpable fracture gap • Painfully limited knee extension • Hemarthrosis • Feeling of instability.

▶ **Treatment options**
Conservative treatment: For nondisplaced fractures (fissure, longitudinal fracture, subaponeurotic fracture) • Immobilization in cylinder cast for 4 weeks.
Surgical treatment: For displaced or transverse fractures • Tension-band wiring (possibly combined with cerclage wiring) to counteract the tensile force of the quadriceps femoris and bring the fragments together under compression • Lag screw fixation in longitudinal and oblique fractures • Comminuted fractures may be managed using Kirschner wires, circumferential and figure-of-eight cerclage wiring, or resorbable suture material via drilling canals • As a last resort, patellectomy • Postoperative early mobilization.

Fig. 9.25 a, b
Transverse fracture
of the patella.
a AP and **b** lateral
radiographs of the
patella.

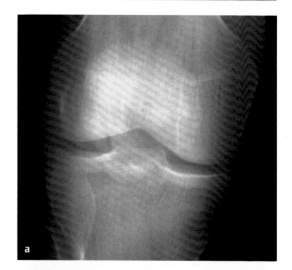

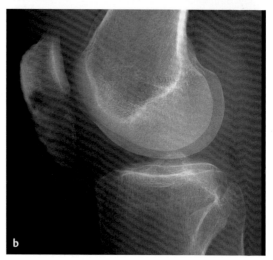

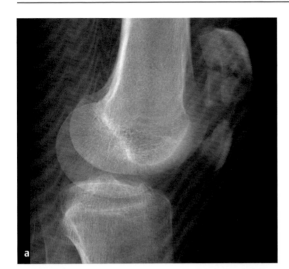

Fig. 9.26 a, b
Comminuted fracture of the patella. **a** AP and **b** lateral radiographs. Stellate fracture with dehiscence of fragments proximally and distally.

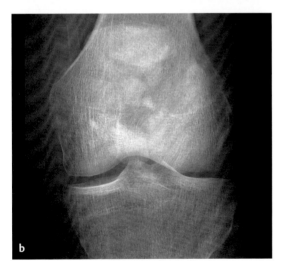

▶ **Course and prognosis**

Very good outcome in 70% ● In 30% weight-bearing-related or constant pain, degenerative joint changes, and chronic irritation with diminished strength and function ● Poorer outcome associated with comminuted and distal transverse fractures.

▶ **What does the clinician want to know?**

Fracture type with or without displacement.

Differential Diagnosis

Bipartite or multipartite patella	– Typical location in superolateral portion of the patella – Bony fragments (two or multiple) do not fit exactly together (unlike in a fracture)

Tips and Pitfalls

Missing smaller, nondisplaced fractures, longitudinal fissures, and small detached flakes ● Mistaking a bipartite patella for a fracture.

Selected References

Mellado JM, Ramos A, Salvado E, Camins A, Calmet J, Sauri A. Avulsion fractures and chronic avulsion injuries of the knee: role of MRI Imaging. Eur Radiol 2002; 12(10): 2463–2473

Definition

▶ **Epidemiology**

1% of all fractures • 75–80% affect the lateral tibial plateau (in 50% there are associated lateral meniscus injuries) and 5–10% the medial tibial plateau • 5–10% bicondylar fractures.

▶ **Etiology, pathophysiology, pathogenesis**

50% of patients are pedestrians injured in traffic accidents • Fall with twisting trauma • Often older women (osteoporosis, mainly compression fractures) and young men (sports-related injuries, often split fracture) • Most common pathomechanisms are valgus stress with or without axial compression forces or, in comminuted fractures, vertical compression forces (fall onto an extended leg) • Fractures of the medial tibial plateau are caused by higher-energy trauma than lateral fractures • Lateral tibial plateau has smaller transverse surface of trabeculae than medial tibial plateau.

Schatzker classification:

– Type I: split fracture of the lateral tibial plateau without depression (mainly in younger patients).

– Type II: split fracture with displacement (dislocation) of lateral articular surface (mainly in older patients with osteoporosis).

– Type III: depression of the lateral tibial plateau without a split fracture through the articular surface.

– Type IV: split fracture of the medial tibial plateau with or without depression.

– Type V: split fracture through medial and lateral tibial plateau.

– Type VI: dissociation of tibial plateau from the underlying metaphysis/diaphysis (massive trauma).

Imaging Signs

▶ **Modality of choice**

Radiography • CT.

▶ **Radiographic findings**

AP and lateral radiographs • Lateral view with horizontal beam (cross-table view) • Oblique views • Follow-up radiographs to monitor healing (look out for loss of reduction) • Path of fracture line • Joint effusion • If lipohemarthrosis is present, cross-table view reveals fat–fluid levels within effusion due to separation of marrow fat (radiotransparent) from heavy blood components.

▶ **CT findings**

For definitive diagnosis with indeterminate radiographs and for surgical planning • Optimal visualization of articular surface depression, split fractures, and bony avulsions.

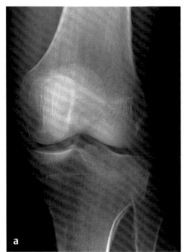

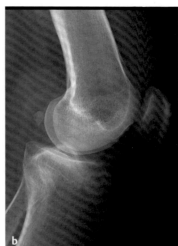

Fig. 9.27 a–c   Lateral tibial plateau fracture involving the intercondylar region. **a** AP and **b** lateral radiographs of the left knee as well as CT reconstruction (**c**). Trabecular compression with a depression in the lateral articular surface (**a, c**) and a fracture line in the metaphysis (**b**).

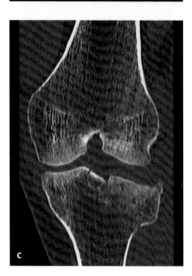

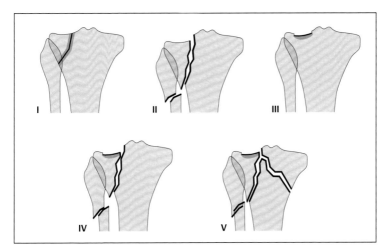

Fig. 9.28 Classification of tibial plateau fractures.

I   Nondisplaced fracture.

II Depression fracture.

III Compression fracture.

IV Compression/depression fracture.

V Bicondylar fracture.

Clinical Aspects

▶ **Typical presentation**

Painfully limited range of motion ● Tenderness ● Soft-tissue swelling ● Hematoma (hemarthrosis almost always present) ● Often associated lesions of internal knee structures.

▶ **Treatment options**

Treatment goals are to establish joint congruence, mechanical axis and joint stability, and to ensure early mobilization.

Conservative treatment: For stable, nondisplaced split fractures ● Plaster cast for 3–4 weeks ● Subsequent physical therapy ● Full weight bearing after 2–3 months.

Surgical treatment: For unstable, displaced fractures • Open reduction • Reconstruction of articular surface • Screw or plate fixation • Larger (metaphyseal) fragments act as key fragments toward which smaller fragments may be oriented • Goal is management with minimal soft-tissue trauma:

– Simple split fracture: screw fixation.
– Condylar fracture: plate fixation with T buttress plate.
– Comminuted fracture: external fixation, perhaps hybrid external fixation.
– Compression/depression fracture: elevation and graft underlay of the depression (if step-off 2 mm or greater) and plate fixation with T plate.

Postoperative early functional mobilization, physical therapy, and use of mobilizing rehabilitation device.

▶ **Course and prognosis**

Most common delayed complications are secondary arthritis due to axial malalignment and joint incongruity • Pseudarthrosis • Osteonecrosis • Instability • Limited range of motion • Prognosis worsens with increasing fracture severity, pre-existing osteopenia, and extent of (traumatic or surgical) soft-tissue damage.

▶ **What does the clinician want to know?**

Detection of fracture • Fracture location • Degree of displacement • Rule out associated injuries of the capsule–ligament complex.

Differential Diagnosis

After ruling out bony lesions, injuries involving the capsule–ligament complex should be precisely diagnosed on MRI • Fractures of other bones at the knee joint.

Tips and Pitfalls

Missing a fracture radiographically if there is no fragment dehiscence • Lipohemarthrosis (fat–fluid levels) may be a sign of fracture • Missing eminence avulsion or fibular head fracture (often associated with instability).

Selected References

Barrow BA, Fajman WA, Parker LM, et al. Tibial plateau fractures: evaluation with MR imaging. Radiographics 1994; 14(3): 553–559

Kode L, Lieberman JM, Motta AO. Evaluation of tibial plateau fractures: efficacy of MR imaging compared with CT. AJR Am J Roentgenol 1994; 163(1): 141–147

Luria S, Liebergall M, Elishoov O, Kandel L, Mattan Y. Osteoporotic tibia plateau fractures: an underestimated cause of knee pain in the elderly. Am J Orthop 2005; 34(3): 186–188

Fractures and Dislocations

Definition

▸ **Epidemiology**
Second most common fracture in humans after distal radius fracture.

▸ **Etiology, pathophysiology, pathogenesis**
Twisting (sprain) injury while walking or running ● Impact of talus against the ankle mortise resulting in fracture of the medial and/or lateral malleolus.

Imaging Signs

▸ **Modality of choice**
Radiographs of ankle joint in two planes (AP and lateral views with 15–20° internal rotation of midfoot/forefoot) ● Presurgical CT in complex fractures.

▸ **Radiographic/CT findings**
AO/Danis-Weber classification based on syndesmosis (just above joint space):
  – Weber A fracture: 10–20% ● Distal fibula fracture below the syndesmosis ● Intact syndesmosis ● Usually supination trauma with adducted foot.
  – Weber B fracture: 45–75% ● Distal fibula fracture at the level of the syndesmosis ● Syndesmosis may be either intact or torn ● Supination or pronation trauma with externally rotated/abducted foot.
  – Weber C fracture: 7–19% ● Fibula fracture above the syndesmosis ● Syndesmosis is always torn ● Rupture of the interosseous membrane extending to the fracture line.
  – Usually pronation trauma with externally rotated foot.
Syndesmotic injury is likely if the joint space between the medial malleolus and trochlea of the talus is widened (wider than between tibia and talus) or if the talus is incongruent and laterally displaced (perpendicular line from longitudinal tibial axis does not intersect midpoint of trochlea).
Possible associated injuries: Oblique shear fracture of the medial malleolus and/or posterior border of the distal tibia ("Volkmann triangle") ● Shear fracture of anterior border of distal tibia ● Coronal fracture line (Tillaux fracture) ● Medial collateral ligament rupture ● Osteochondral fracture of the talus ● Fracture-dislocation.
Maisonneuve fracture: Proximal fibular fracture ● Rupture of syndesmosis ● Longitudinal rupture of interosseous membrane extending to fracture (usually sprain injury).
Trimalleolar fracture: Bimalleolar fracture with avulsion of the posterior border of the tibia ("Volkmann triangle") ● There may also be dislocation of the trochlea of talus (fracture-dislocation).
Tibial pilon fracture: Vertically oriented fracture of the distal tibia ● Usually severe impaction trauma (extra-articular, partial articular fracture, complete articular fracture).
Triplane fracture: Fracture in three planes ● Sagittally through epiphysis ● Horizontally through tibia ● Coronally through metaphysis.

▸ **CT findings**
In complex fractures (e.g., trimalleolar, tibial pilon fracture, triplane, or Tillaux), especially if displacement is present.

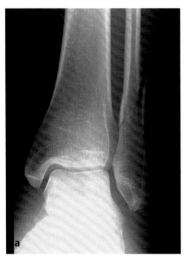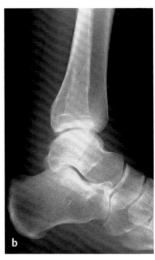

Fig. 9.29 a, b AP (**a**) and lateral (**b**) radiographs of an ankle fracture in a 35-year-old woman with a Weber C fracture.

▶ **MRI findings**
To clarify the presence of a ligamentous lesion or ruptured syndesmosis ● In axial and angulated T2-weighted images, disruption of ligament with fluid signal ● There may be an osteochondral fragment (flake).

Clinical Aspects

▶ **Typical presentation**
Pain ● Swelling about the ankle joint ● Inability to bear weight.
▶ **Treatment options**
Conservative treatment: For Weber A fractures and nondisplaced Weber B fractures ● Short leg cast for 6 weeks.
Surgical treatment: For Weber C fractures and displaced Weber B fractures (fragment displacement exceeding 2 mm) ● Also for Maisonneuve, bimalleolar, trimalleolar, and medial malleolar fractures ● Plate fixation of fibula ● Syndesmotic screw between distal fibula and tibia ● For fractures of the medial malleolus, tension banding or lag screw fixation ● Operative intervention if Volkmann triangle involves more than 1 cm of articular portion of tibia.
▶ **Course and prognosis**
Prognosis usually good ● Possibility of secondary post-traumatic arthritis, especially in tibial pilon fractures.
▶ **What does the clinician want to know?**
Classification of fracture ● Displacement ● Avulsion involving ankle mortise as a sign of joint instability?

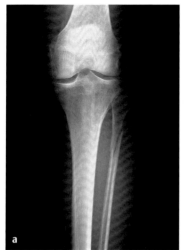
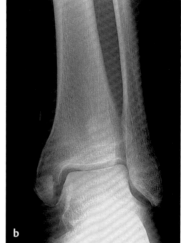

Fig. 9.30 a, b   An 83-year-old man after a fall. **a** AP radiograph of the lower left leg and knee joint; **b** AP radiograph of the left ankle joint. Maisonneuve fracture (high Weber C fracture) and fracture of the medial malleolus.

Differential Diagnosis

Lateral collateral ligament rupture without fracture	– Virtually impossible to distinguish clinically due to marked soft-tissue swelling and hematomas. Always obtain radiographs!

Tips and Pitfalls

Missing a proximal fibular lesion (Maisonneuve fracture); the proximal fibula should therefore always be tested for pain on palpation.

Selected References

Beltran J, Shankman S. MR imaging of bone lesions of the ankle and foot. Magn Reson Imaging Clin North Am 2001; 9(3): 553–566

Campbell SE. MRI of sports injuries of the ankle. Clin Sports Med 2006; 25(4): 727–762

Harper MC. Ankle fracture classification systems: a case for integration of the Lauge-Hansen and AO-Danis-Weber schemes. Foot Ankle 1992; 13(7): 404–407

Kor A, Saltzman AT, Wempe PD. Medial malleolar stress fractures. Literature review, diagnosis, and treatment [review]. J Am Podiatr Med Assoc 2003; 93(4): 292–297

Muthukumar T, Butt SH, Cassar-Pullicino VN. Stress fractures and related disorders in foot and ankle: plain films, scintigraphy, CT, and MR imaging. Semin Musculoskelet Radiol 2005; 9(3): 210–226

Prokuski LJ, Saltzman CL. Challenging fractures of the foot and ankle. Radiol Clin North Am 1997; 35(3): 655–670

Definition

▶ **Epidemiology**

Most common fracture of tarsal bones (60%) • In two-thirds of patients, additional involvement of talocalcaneal joint • Bilateral in 10% • Intra-articular fracture in 80% • Calcaneocuboid joint involved in 50% • Open fracture in 2%.

▶ **Etiology, pathophysiology, pathogenesis**

Fall from a great height with axial compression of the heel • Motor vehicle accidents • Impact against hard surface during running or jumping • Force of impact compresses the harder talus against the relatively soft calcaneus • Stress fractures may be seen in athletes • Rarely, pathologic fracture associated with cysts/lipomas • NB: 10–20% of patients have additional compression fractures in the thoracolumbar spine.

Fracture line is usually vertical and passes through the central talus • Depending on the position of the foot, secondary fracture lines are as follows:

– In the dorsiflexed foot, depression of posterior articular facet into the main posterolateral fragment (joint-depression fracture).

– In the plantar-flexed foot, horizontal fracture line through the calcaneal tuberosity with rotation of this fragment.

Subdivided into peripheral and central fractures (usually involving the talocalcaneal joint) • Sanders classification of central fractures (based on CT findings):

– Type I: nondisplaced fracture.

– Type II: displaced fracture, two-fragment or split fracture.

– Type III: displaced fracture, three-fragment or compression/split fracture.

– Type IV: displaced fracture, four-fragment or comminuted fracture.

Peripheral fractures: isolated fracture of the anterior talar articular surface, sustentaculum tali, or calcaneal tuberosity, as well as avulsion fractures (beak fractures produced by avulsion of Achilles tendon attachment).

Imaging Signs

▶ **Modality of choice**

Radiography • CT.

▶ **Radiographic findings**

Radiographs of the ankle joint in two planes • Axial calcaneal view • Classic, and sometimes only, radiographic sign is a decreased Boehler angle of less than 20° (physiologic angle is 35°) on lateral projections • Angle may be negative in patients with severe compression • Best assessment of calcaneal widening (normal width is 30–35 mm) is on axial views • Widening may also be visible on AP ankle view if lateral calcaneal margin projects beyond the tip of the lateral malleolus.

▶ **CT findings**

Precise evaluation of fracture type and surgical planning • Evaluation of talonavicular and calcaneocuboid joints as well as sustentaculum tali on axial images • Depiction of posterior facet on coronal images • Evaluation of fracture type and fragments in comminuted fractures • Surgical planning (key fragment is talocal-

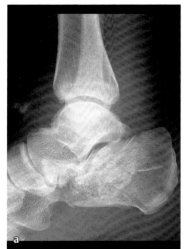

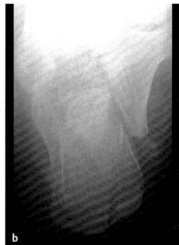

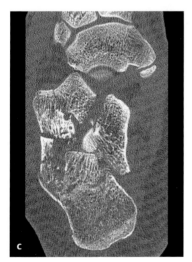

Fig. 9.31 a–d   Comminuted fracture of the calcaneus. **a** Lateral and **b** axial radiographs of the right calcaneus. **c** Coronal and **d** sagittal CT. Decreased Boehler angle (**a, d**) and widened calcaneus (**b, c**).

caneal joint with sustentaculum tali since it usually does not change position relative to the talus).

▶ **MRI findings**

If stress fracture is suspected despite apparently normal radiographic findings.

Fig. 9.31 d

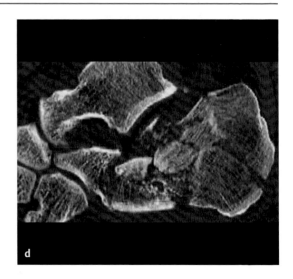

Clinical Aspects

▶ **Typical presentation**

Swelling ● Hematoma ● Deformity ● Painfully limited range of motion ● Tenderness ● Pain on percussion ● Compression pain.

▶ **Treatment options**

Goal of treatment: reconstruction of articular surfaces restoring form and function.

Conservative treatment: For all fractures in which malalignment does not mandate reduction.

Surgical treatment: Beak fractures require lag screw fixation ● Relative surgical indication for intra-articular fractures with compression and displaced fractures ● Open reduction with plate/screw fixation ● External fixation.

▶ **Course and prognosis**

Main prognostic factor is degree of intra-articular displacement ● Good long-term prognosis in 90% of extra-articular and nondisplaced intra-articular fractures ● Injuries with joint damage are always affected by post-traumatic arthritis.

▶ **What does the clinician want to know?**

Size and location of main fragments ● Widening, shortening, flattening, and varus-producing position of the calcaneus ● Involvement and damage of articular surfaces ● Involvement of calcaneocuboid joint.

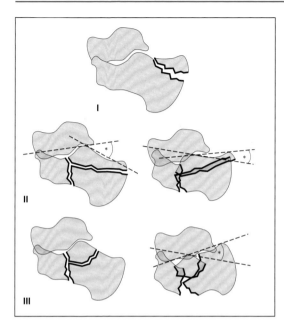

Fig. 9.32 Varieties of central, primary vertical calcaneal fracture lines and Boehler angle (*).

I   Beak fracture, peripheral type.
II Beak fracture, tongue-type.
III Beak fracture, joint-depression type.

Differential Diagnosis

Calcaneus secundarius	– Accessory ossicle
	– Patient history
	– Sclerotic border
Stress fracture	– Patient history
	– Vertical fracture line perpendicular to posterosuperior cortex

Tips and Pitfalls

Missing a nondisplaced fracture.

Selected References

Daftary A, Haims AH, Baumgaertner MR. Fractures of the calcaneus: a review with emphasis on CT. Radiographics 2005; 25(5): 1215–1226

Lim EV, Leung JP. Complications of intraarticular calcaneal fractures. Clin Orthop Relat Res 2001; (391): 7–16

Maskill JD, Bohay DR, Anderson JG. Calcaneus fractures: a review article. Foot Ankle Clin 2005; 10(3): 463–489

Definition

▶ **Epidemiology**

Most common fracture of the midfoot ● Men and women equally affected ● Avulsion fracture of the fifth metatarsal tuberosity in 90% of cases.

▶ **Etiology, pathophysiology, pathogenesis**

Acute trauma with forced supination ● Avulsion fracture mediated by lateral portion of plantar aponeurosis and the tendon of the peroneus brevis ● Usually only minimal displacement (< 2 mm).

Jones fracture: Near the base (within 1.5 cm of joint line), on the proximal shaft ● Usually caused by direct trauma.

Stress fracture: Typically more than 1.5 cm distal to the joint line ● Overuse or decreased stability of the bone ● Impaired circulation may be responsible for high rate of pseudarthroses.

Torg classification system:

- Type I: sharp fracture margins ● No displacement of fragments ● No sclerosis ● No periosteal reaction.
- Type II: dehiscence of fracture gap ● Periosteal reaction ● Variable degree of sclerosis (delayed union).
- Type III: dehiscence of fracture gap ● Periosteal reaction ● Clearly sclerotic fracture margins (nonunion).

Imaging Signs

▶ **Modality of choice**

Radiography ● Perhaps CT.

▶ **Radiographic findings**

Radiographs of forefoot in two planes ● Usually horizontal radiolucent line at the base of the fifth metatarsal bone running perpendicular to its longitudinal axis ● Cortical disruption ● In nondisplaced impacted fractures, radiodense line at corresponding site ● Soft-tissue swelling on lateral margin of foot ● In stress fractures, additional periosteal reaction and variable amount of sclerosis.

▶ **CT findings**

In severe trauma for evaluation of involvement of the joint and of Lisfranc's joint.

Clinical Aspects

▶ **Typical presentation**

Pain ● Swelling along the lateral margin of the foot (distinguish from ankle joint trauma with swelling of lateral malleolus) ● Inability to bear weight.

▶ **Treatment options**

- Torg I fracture: usually conservative.
- Torg II fracture: conservative or operative.
- Torg III fracture: operative (Kirschner wire, intramedullary screw fixation).

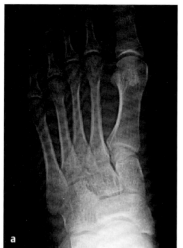

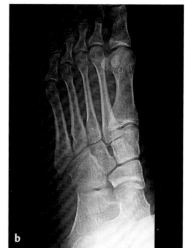

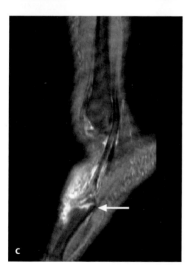

Fig. 9.33 a–c   Avulsion fracture of the base of the fifth metatarsal bone.
a DP radiograph of the foot. The barely discernible fracture line can be seen running perpendicular to the longitudinal axis.
b Oblique view. The fracture line is much more easily identified.
c Oblique sagittal fat-saturated proton density-weighted MRI. Avulsion fracture (arrow) with involvement of the peroneal tendon, which is torn.

▶ **Course and prognosis**

Prognosis good if diagnosed early with adequate relief of weight bearing ● Jones fracture has a tendency to pseudarthrosis and is thus often managed with screw fixation.

▶ **What does the clinician want to know?**

Fragment displacement ● Articular involvement ● Rule out ankle fracture.

Differential Diagnosis

Ankle fracture	– Typical radiographic findings
Epiphyseal plate at base of fifth metatarsal	– Parallel to longitudinal axis, does not extend to tarsometatarsal joint
	– Epiphyseal ossific nucleus is curved rather than wedge-shaped and recognizable as a distinct bony element in patients aged 9–14 years
Os peroneum, os vesalianum	– Rounded shape
	– Cortical margin

Tips and Pitfalls

False-positive diagnosis of a fracture in patients in whom the epiphyseal plate is still open.

Selected References

Fetzer GB, Wright RW. Metatarsal shaft fractures and fractures of the proximal fifth metatarsal. Clin Sports Med 2006; 25(1): 139–150

Lawrence SJ, Botte MJ. Jones' fractures and related fractures of the proximal fifth metatarsal. Foot Ankle 1993; 14(6): 358–365

Nunley JA. Fractures of the base of the fifth metatarsal: the Jones fracture. Orthop Clin North Am 2001; 32(1): 171–180

Pao DG, Keats TE, Dussault RG. Avulsion fracture of the base of the fifth metatarsal not seen on conventional radiography of the foot: the need for an additional projection. AJR Am J Roentgenol 2000; 175(2): 549–552

Stewart IM. Jones's fracture: fracture of base of fifth metatarsal. Clin Orthop 1960; 16: 190–8

Stoller D. Ankle and Foot. Magnetic Resonance Imaging in Orthopaedics and Sports Medicine. 2nd ed. Philadelphia: Lippincott, Williams & Wilkins, 1996: 568–569

Torg JS, Balduini FC, Zelko RR, Pavlov H, Peff TC, Das M. Fractures of the base of the fifth metatarsal distal to the tuberosity. Classification and guidelines for non-surgical and surgical management. J Bone Joint Surg Am 1984; 66(2): 209–214

Definition

▶ **Epidemiology**
Nondisplaced fracture that is undetectable on radiographs despite correct imaging technique ● 2–9% of femoral neck fractures are occult ● 15% of scaphoid fractures are occult.

▶ **Etiology, pathophysiology, pathogenesis**
As for evident fractures.

Imaging Signs

▶ **Modality of choice**
MRI ● CT ● Nuclear medicine (in older patients, not positive until after 1–3 days).

▶ **CT findings**
High-resolution spiral CT ● Fracture line, cortical step-off, cortical disruption, or trabecular radiodensities ● Especially for imaging of wrist, tarsal bones, and spine.

▶ **MRI findings**
Sensitivity is 93% ● Specificity is 95% ● On T1-weighted and T2-weighted sequences, linear or bandlike decreased signal intensity in the bone marrow extending to the cortex ● On T2-weighted or STIR sequences, perifocal edema ● On T2-weighted images, fracture line is hypointense due to trabecular compression ● Central linear hyperintensity is evident with widened fracture gap ● On GE sequences, susceptibility effects give rise to variously large signal voids ● Associated soft-tissue injuries may be found (hematoma, muscle contusion) ● There may be epiphyseal involvement ● Especially in the pelvis, MRI may depict fractures that are much more extensive than suspected.

Clinical Aspects

▶ **Typical presentation**
E.g., femoral neck fracture: unlike usual patient history (fall with subsequent hip or knee pain; swollen, shortened, abducted, externally rotated lower extremity), only mild symptoms on passive motion ● In nondisplaced fractures weight bearing may even be possible.
E.g., scaphoid fracture: tenderness over anatomic snuffbox and scaphoid tubercle ● Axial compression pain along index finger.

▶ **Treatment options**
As for evident fractures.

▶ **Course and prognosis**
Goals of early diagnosis are reduction of comorbidity (e.g., by immobilization), prevention of secondary displacement, and prevention of pseudarthrosis.

▶ **What does the clinician want to know?**
Diagnosis ● Evaluation of fracture consolidation over the course of healing (especially CT) ● Rule out necrosis.

Fractures and Dislocations

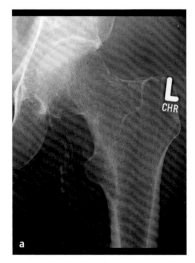 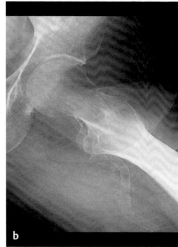

Fig. 9.34 a–d Fall onto the left hip.
a AP and **b** lateral radiographs of the left hip. No visible fracture.

Differential Diagnosis

Bone contusion	– Signal alterations on MRI resembling bone marrow edema
	– No fracture line

Tips and Pitfalls

Failing to follow up with (sectional) imaging studies when initial radiographic findings are negative.

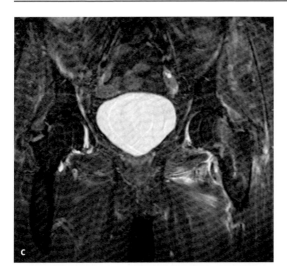

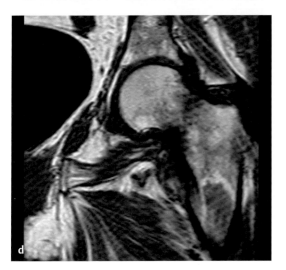

c Coronal and **d** sagittal MRI. Fracture lines through the femoral neck and involving the greater trochanter.

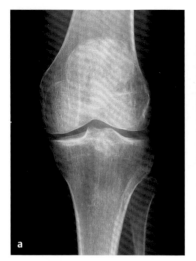 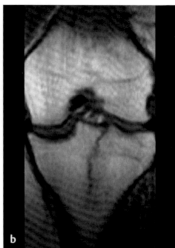

Fig. 9.35 a, b   Pain in left knee joint after a fall.
a AP radiograph of left knee. Unremarkable findings.
b MRI. Sagittal fracture line in tibial plateau.

Selected References

Deutsch AL, Mink JH, Shellock FG. Magnetic resonance imaging of injuries to bone and articular cartilage. Emphasis on radiographically occult abnormalities. Orthop Rev 1990; 19(1): 66–75

Memarsadeghi M, Breitenseher MJ, Schaefer-Prokop C, et al. Occult scaphoid fractures: comparison of multidetector CT and MR imaging—initial experience. Radiology 2006; 240(1):169–176

Mittal RL, Dargan SK. Occult scaphoid fracture: a diagnostic enigma. J Orthop Trauma 1989; 3(4): 306–308

Newhouse KE, el-Khoury GY, Buckwalter JA. Occult sacral fractures in osteopenic patients. J Bone Joint Surg Am 1992; 74(10): 1472–1477

Peh WC, Gilula LA, Wilson AJ. Detection of occult wrist fractures by magnetic resonance imaging. Clin Radiol 1996; 51(4): 285–292

Perron AD, Miller MD, Brady WJ (2002) Orthopedic pitfalls in the ED: radiographically occult hip fracture. Am J Emerg Med 2002; 20(3):234–237

Rizzo M, Shin AY (2006) Treatment of acute scaphoid fractures in the athlete. Curr Sports Med Rep 2006; 5(5):242–248

Rizzo PF, Gould ES, Lyden JP, Asnis SE. Diagnosis of occult fractures about the hip. Magnetic resonance imaging compared with bone-scanning. J Bone Joint Surg Am 1993; 75(3): 395–401

Definition

▶ **Epidemiology**
"Stress fracture" is a generic term for fatigue and insufficiency fractures ● Lower extremities and pelvis are most usually affected ● Up to 20% of all injuries in sports medicine are stress fractures ● Competitive sports and running are responsible for 70% of all stress fractures ● Osteoporosis (both primary and secondary) is a central feature of insufficiency fractures.

▶ **Etiology, pathophysiology, pathogenesis**
Imbalance between bone formation and resorption with disproportionate increase in osteoclast activity ● Trabecular, and later cortical, microfractures ● Attempted repair by the body with periosteal new bone formation.
Fatigue fracture: Repetitive inappropriate submaximal stress of normal bone ● Stress reaction: no manifest fracture.
Insufficiency fracture: Physiologic stress of bone tissue with low elasticity or diminished mineral salt content (e.g., in osteoporosis, Paget disease, or osteomalacia) ● When malignancy is present, also referred to as pathologic fracture.

Imaging Signs

▶ **Modality of choice**
Radiography ● MRI ● Nuclear medicine ● CT.

▶ **Radiographic findings**
Low sensitivity (15%) in early stages ● Increased radiotransparency, indistinct cortex, and lamellar periosteal reaction or callus formation may not be present initially ● Most valuable early radiographic sign is periosteal reaction ● Marked solid or lamellar periosteal reaction, fracture line, and callus formation often take weeks to appear ● Fracture line subsequently disappears as a sign of healing.

▶ **CT findings**
In cortical stress fractures, CT may not demonstrate fracture lines or periosteal/endosteal new bone formation until after 2–3 weeks ● Stress fractures involving trabecular bone exhibit diffuse sclerosis with blunt margins (endosteal callus, trabecular condensation) ● In more long-standing sacral insufficiency fractures, fracture margins are rounded and sclerotic ● Negative density values are key to differentiating osteoporotic and tumor-related fractures ● Longitudinal stress fracture of the tibia (up to 10%) can aid diagnosis.

▶ **Nuclear medicine**
Very high sensitivity ● Lower specificity than radiography (differential diagnoses include tumor, infection, bone infarct, periostitis) ● Intense, focally increased tracer uptake 6–72 hours after trauma (linear or spindle-shaped) ● Given normal radiographic findings, can distinguish between osseous and extraosseous lesions ● In early stages, slightly elevated tracer uptake which increases notably in later stages ● In bilateral insufficiency sacral fracture, Honda sign: H-shaped tracer accumulation.

Fig. 9.36 Calcaneal fatigue fracture. Having stopped running for several years, the patient experienced heel pain upon starting again. Lateral radiograph of the calcaneus shows a linear radiodensity (arrow) perpendicular to the superoposterior calcaneus.

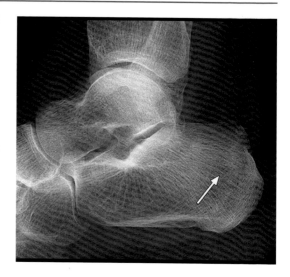

▶ **MRI findings**

Highest sensitivity on fat-saturated T2-weighted and STIR sequences ● Assists diagnosis when radiographic findings are negative.

Stress reaction: Early increased signal (STIR, T2-weighted TSE sequences) ● Signal intensity resembling that of bone marrow.

Stress fracture: Signal intensity resembling that of bone marrow ● On all sequences: hypointense fracture line (usually perpendicular to the cortex, though in rare situations in the tibia may be parallel to the adjacent cortex) ● Widened fracture line may produce centrally increased signal intensity ● Often prominent periosteal reaction with extensive edema and contrast enhancement ● As healing progresses, callus formation and diminished evidence of above-mentioned changes ● Typical butterfly appearance of edema in bilateral sacral insufficiency fractures.

Clinical Aspects

▶ **Typical presentation**

Diagnosis mainly based on patient history ● Gradual onset of symptoms ● Related to unusual level of physical activity (change of routine/duration) ● Worsening with continued physical activity ● Improvement at rest ● Osteoporosis is important etiological factor.

Sites of predilection: proximal tibia, navicular (foot), calcaneus, second and third metatarsal bones, femoral neck, and pelvis ● Pelvic fractures mainly involve bilateral stress fractures of sacrum, femoral neck fractures, fractures of the ilium

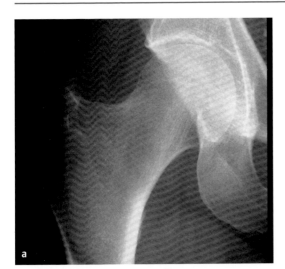

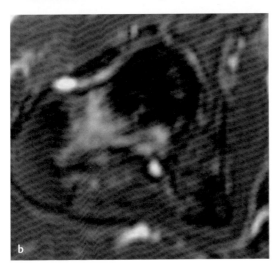

Fig. 9.37 a–d
Stress fracture after
rapidly increasing
the level of intensity
of jogging activity.
Pain in right hip
joint.
a AP radiograph of
the right hip shows
unremarkable find-
ings.
b MRI. Edema.

c Repeat radiograph 1 month later. Sclerotic area that extends to the cortex. No evidence of cortical fracture.
d Follow-up CT after 2 months. Small cortical fracture and periosteal reaction.

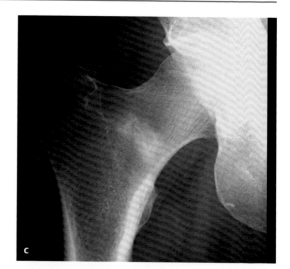

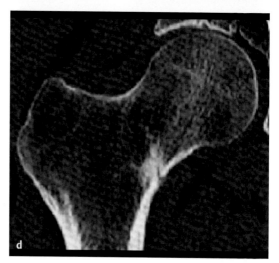

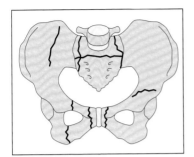

Fig. 9.38 Typical orientations of stress fracture lines in the pelvis.

above the acetabulum, and pubic bone fractures • Especially in children, an L4 or L5 pars interarticularis fracture is possible.

▶ **Treatment options**

Reduce weight bearing • Cast • Analgesics.

▶ **Course and prognosis**

Good prognosis for stress reaction if treated early • Good prognosis for established fractures if sufficiently immobilized • NB: sacral fractures often involve pseudarthrosis.

▶ **What does the clinician want to know?**

Early diagnosis and exclusion of differential diagnoses (e.g., tumor or inflammation).

Differential Diagnosis

Key aspects in establishing diagnosis are patient history, location, and combination of periosteal reaction and linear area of sclerosis oriented perpendicularly to the cortex.

Osteoid osteoma	– Pain worsens at night – Pain responds well to aspirin – Nidus, marked sclerosis
Chronic sclerosing osteomyelitis (Garré osteomyelitis)	– Sclerotic appearance – Often no increased radiotransparency on radiographs – More extensive involvement – No changes apparent over period of weeks
Osteomalacia	– Looser zones of transformation – Rugger jersey spine – Coarse bone texture – Deformity of long tubular bones – Chronic renal insufficiency (renal osteodystrophy)
Bone metastasis	– Insufficiency fractures of sacrum/pelvis often related to underlying malignancy

Osteogenic sarcoma	– Usually metaphyseal
	– Moth-eaten appearance
	– Spiculated/thin lamellar periosteal reaction
	– Codman triangle possible
Ewing sarcoma	– Diaphysis of long tubular bones
	– Osteolytic destruction
Shin splints	– Periostitis of posteromedial tibia at junction between middle and distal third
	– Diffuse tracer uptake on bone scans

Tips and Pitfalls

Missing a sacral insufficiency fracture on radiographs • Mistaking a stress fracture for tumor or infection because of marked periosteal reactions.

Selected References

Anderson MW. Imaging of upper extremity stress fractures in the athlete. Clin Sports Med 2006; 25(3): 489–504, vii

Bergman AG, Fredericson M. MR imaging of stress reactions, muscle injuries, and other overuse injuries in runners. Magn Reson Imaging Clin North Am 1999; 7(1): 151–174, ix

Muthukumar T, Butt SH, Cassar-Pullicino VN. Stress fractures and related disorders in foot and ankle: plain films, scintigraphy, CT, and MR imaging. Semin Musculoskelet Radiol 2005; 9(3): 210–226

Wall J, Feller JF. Imaging of stress fractures in runners. Clin Sports Med 2006; 25(4): 781–802

Weishaupt D, Schweitzer ME. MR imaging of the foot and ankle: patterns of bone marrow signal abnormalities. Eur Radiol 2002; 12(2): 416–426

Definition

▶ **Epidemiology**
Failure of bones to unite 8 months after fracture • Predilection for diaphyseal region • Commonly affects scaphoid, tibial shaft, femoral neck.

▶ **Etiology, pathophysiology, pathogenesis**
Causes:
 – Inadequate immobilization.
 – No contact between fragments: soft-tissue interposition • Distraction due to tensile forces or osteosynthetic devices • Malalignment • Secondary dislocation • Extensive loss of bone tissue.
 – Inadequate/disrupted blood supply: damage to supplying vessels • Periosteal injury • Osteonecrosis.
 – Infection: osteomyelitis • Bone destruction and sequestration • Osteolysis • Implant loosening.
Instead of bony union at the fracture site, the bones are merely joined by fibrous tissue.
Classified as:
 – Hypertrophic (reactive) nonunion: usually due to inadequate immobilization.
 – Atrophic (nonreactive) nonunion: with extensive bony defects or inadequate blood supply.
 – Nonunion with infection.

Imaging Signs

▶ **Modality of choice**
Radiography • CT • Possibly nuclear medicine.

▶ **Radiographic findings**
Fracture gap still evident after 6 months • Rounded fragment ends with smooth margins • It may be possible to demonstrate fragments rubbing against each other.
 – Hypertrophic nonunion: excessive new bone formation with expanded and sclerotic fracture ends (elephant's foot).
 – Atrophic nonunion: no callus formation, sclerotic margins at fracture line.
 – Infected nonunion: distinguish between active or and inactive infection • Inactive infection: cortex is irregular and expanded, spongy bone exhibits reactive sclerosis, and there is marked periosteal new bone formation • Active infection: bone destruction, sequestra, and soft-tissue swelling.

▶ **CT findings**
Helpful in evaluating possible discreet (masked on radiographs) callus formation in complex anatomical regions, e.g., wrist or foot • Initial osteophytes near fracture site • Resorption zones.

▶ **Nuclear medicine**
Hypertrophic nonunion: fragment ends are vascular, hence increased tracer uptake • Atrophic nonunion: blood supply is typically poor, hence low tracer uptake.

Fig. 9.39 a, b
Scaphoid
pseudarthrosis.
a PA radiograph of
the wrist showing
delayed healing
with resorption and
sclerotic areas
around the fracture
site. Dehiscence of
the fracture gap.
b Pseudarthrosis/
nonunion with car-
pal instability and
secondary degener-
ative changes af-
fecting the radio-
scaphoid joint.

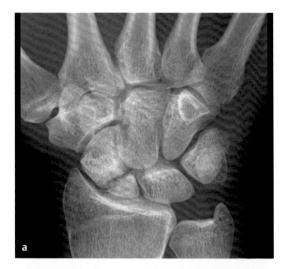

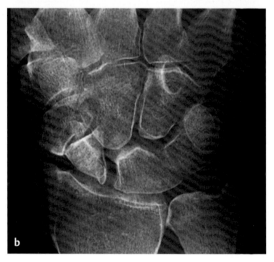

Clinical Aspects

▸ **Typical presentation**
Feeling of instability ● Pathologic mobility in severe cases ● Pain ● Swelling ● Inability to bear weight.

▸ **Treatment options**
   – Hypertrophic nonunion: stabilization ● Intramedullary nails ● Plate fixation ● External fixation.
   – Atrophic nonunion: rigid fixation ● Decortication ● Autologous bone transplant.
   – Infected nonunion: stabilization ● Radical resection of infected tissue ● Subsequent spongiosaplasty.

▸ **Course and prognosis**
Good prognosis in hypertrophic nonunion ● Prognosis usually unfavorable in infected nonunion.

▸ **What does the clinician want to know?**
Confirm diagnosis ● Signs of infection ● Classification.

Differential Diagnosis

Accessory ossicle	– Independent bone
	– Commonly found at typical site
	– No identifiable congruence with adjacent bones

Tips and Pitfalls

Failure to detect abnormal fracture healing and perform follow-up studies for further assessment.

Selected References

Coblenz G, Christopoulos G, Frohner S, Kalb KH, Schmitt R. Scaphoid fracture and nonunion: current status of radiological diagnostics [in German]. Radiologe 2006; 46(8): 664, 666–676

Ekkernkamp A, Muhr G, Josten C. Infected pseudarthrosis [review, in German]. Unfallchirurg 1996; 99(12): 914–924

Ruter A, Mayr E. Pseudarthrosis [review, in German]. Chirurg 1999; 70(11): 1239–1245

Shalom A, Khermosh O, Wientroub S. The natural history of congenital pseudarthrosis of the clavicle. J Bone Joint Surg Br 1994; 76(5): 846–847

Singh HP, Forward D, Davis TR et al. Partial union of acute scaphoid fractures. J Hand Surg Br 2005; 30(5): 440–445

Sloan A, Paton R. Congenital pseudarthrosis of the clavicle: the role of CT-scanning. Acta Orthop Belg 2006; 72(3): 356–358

Page numbers in *italics* refer to
illustrations.

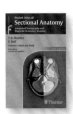
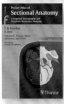
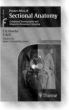
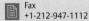 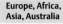